Journey to Equity

JOURNEY TO EQUITY

Strengthening the Profession of Nursing

EDITORS

CAROL SUSAN "SUE" JOHNSON,
PhD, RN, NE-BC, NPD-BC, FAAN

PAMELA S. DICKERSON,
PhD, RN, NPDA-BC®, FAAN

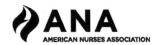

ANA
AMERICAN NURSES ASSOCIATION

About the American Nurses Association
The American Nurses Association (ANA) is the only full-service professional organization representing the interests of the nation's 4.3 million registered nurses through its constituent/state nurses associations and its organizational affiliates. The ANA advances the nursing profession by fostering high standards of nursing practice, promoting the rights of nurses in the workplace, projecting a positive and realistic view of nursing, and by lobbying the Congress and regulatory agencies on health care issues affecting nurses and the public.

American Nurses Association
8515 Georgia Avenue, Suite 400
Silver Spring, MD 20910

Cataloging in Publication data available from the Library of Congress

ISBNs
Print 978-1-947800-85-4
ePDF 978-1-947800-86-1
ePUB 978-1-947800-87-8
Mobi 978-1-947800-88-5

SAN: 851-3481

DEDICATION

This book is dedicated to all future nurses who will truly represent the communities they serve. Our thanks to everyone who collaborated to share their own journeys with us and our readers. The nursing profession can and must lead the way to equity, and we challenge our colleagues to use this book as a template to create a future where equity in health care is truly attainable.

—Carol Susan "Sue" Johnson,
PhD, RN, NE-BC, NPD-BC, FAAN

—Pamela S. Dickerson,
PhD, RN, NPDA-BC', FAAN

CONTENTS

Diversity, Equity, and Inclusion: How Far Have We Really Come?

Launette Woolforde,
EdD, DNP, RN, NEA-BC, NPD-BC, FAAN
Chief Nursing Officer, Northwell Health

D iversity, equity, and inclusion. These terms have increased exponentially in popularity. However, the question remains about how much progress we have truly made in each of these areas. Certainly, as a nation, we are a more diverse population. Equity and inclusion, however . . . well, that journey continues. I find it interesting that "diverse" has now taken on a new definition as a way to identify a person. All too often, when inquiring about whether an individual is a person of color, for example, the substitute question asked is, "Are they diverse?" I am left to wonder when a "diverse" person became a pseudonym for a non-White person. I always thought that being diverse or coming from a diverse background meant you had several different elements such as racial, cultural, or other representations in your background. I question this new definition of diverse, and whether labeling someone who likely already experiences other labels, as diverse, isn't more alienating than anything else. It reminds me of the stores I would visit to purchase personal items. It was always odd to come upon the aisle labeled "ethnic products." Of course, that was the aisle for (usually skin and hair) care products for non-White people who had now been termed "ethnic." Ultimately, the message it sends is that the items for White people are normalized, need no label, and just go in a regular skin and hair care products aisle, and then there's the aisle for the other people. Similarly, there's the concept of nude. I always think of this in relation to pantyhose or shoe shopping. There's not just the difficulty of finding inclusivity in tones, but there's the hijacking of the definition of nude. I've always known nude to be representative of naked or transparent so that nude pantyhose would make my legs appear nude, or without covering. Yet whenever I purchase nude pantyhose, or nude shoes for that matter, I have to ask myself, "Nude according to whom? This is not nude; it's clearly light beige. It's anything but nude." The term "diverse "has become redefined to normalize Whiteness and serves as one of the many reminders in society of hierarchy, power, and inequity that are glaring to those subjected to it daily. Those who are not subjected to those inequities are often oblivious and may even deny its truth or find derogatory names to call those who speak about it.

I am, among other things, a Black woman. In many cases, representation by someone like me helps to create diversity in groups that have been plagued by homogeneity. I think about how often, by virtue of being the only one, the one who brings diversity to the group, I become the representative of my entire race, bearing much more responsibility than anyone else in the group. Nonetheless, this does not make me diverse. I do wonder what it is like to live free of these and so many other daily burdens and just be you. Someone who comes with only favorable preconceived notions, inherent inclusion, and for whom matters like these are mere abject conversation.

To be diverse means to be inclusive or representative of many elements. Diverse is not a person, nor should it become another label for those outside of the mainstream or marginalized groups to bear. Everyone has a hand in diversity. There are those who equate diversity strategies with unfairness, almost like a robbery of opportunity for some. Aiming for diversity does not mean "exclusion of"; it means "more than just." A diverse setting is one where people from a mainstream group are represented along with people from nonmainstream groups. A single person in that group is not the diverse one; it is the presence of varying representations that makes the group diverse.

Health care can represent one of the most inequitable experiences one can have. In March of 1966 at a meeting of the Medical Committee for Human Rights in Chicago, in reference to the disparate medical care received by Black people, Dr. Martin Luther King Jr. stated,

> We are concerned about the constant use of federal funds to support this most notorious expression of segregation. Of all the forms of inequality, injustice in health is the most shocking and the most inhuman because it often results in physical death. (Mt. Vernon Register News, 1966, p. 5)

Healthcare inequities persist today. Communities comprised primarily of people of color are consistently and disproportionately exposed to pollution, environmental hazards, and discriminatory practices that put them at greater risk for almost all illnesses. The age-old pandemic of racism underscores inequities, and its manifestations are heightened in times of crises.

Nurses have a unique opportunity to advocate for equity in care delivery. Nurses collaborate with other members of the care delivery team and contribute to the development and execution of the plan of care. Incorporating equity awareness should be an integral part of our role and practice.

Attention to diversity and inclusiveness exposes the need to examine ourselves and the inclusiveness, or lack thereof, of our settings and of our practice (Woolforde, 2018). Everyone plays a role in the journey to equity, either by actively taking steps toward improvement, by promulgating environments and processes that perpetuate inequity, or through standing by, another mechanism that promulgates inequity but allows the bystander to find ways to absolve themselves of accountability.

So, what are three steps every person can take to help build a healthcare system and an environment that fosters diversity, inclusion, and equity?

Understand Your Community

While there are constants in health care that haven't changed in centuries, such as handwashing as the most effective method to prevent the spread of infection, we have to go beyond the routine and aim to understand the composition and needs of the communities we serve. We must then adjust education and care planning to meet the needs of the community. We should point out and address the disparities and place emphasis on adjusting planning and resources according to these realities in order to achieve optimal wellness. Inequities might be related to language, lack of cultural awareness among staff, lack of cultural awareness integration into the plan of care, and more. Having a diverse workforce that is reflective of the community helps to mitigate these divides. These changes can translate into significant improvements in health outcomes and great satisfaction among those providing care—not just those receiving it.

Educate Yourself

Nurses spend a lot of time educating others. Equally important, however, is educating oneself, not just on the latest in clinical care but on one's own biases or lack of knowledge about the community one serves and how to modify plans and care to address needs. Nurses have the power to design and deliver initiatives that incorporate equity considerations and demonstrate for others across professions how this is done.

Build an Army of Advocates

Nurses interact with a wide variety of care providers at all levels of practice. Role-modeling advocacy practices is an important part of our responsibility. Take a stance on unequal treatment and build an army of people who have learned from you that they, too, must do the same. Trade fear for fearlessness. Advocating for equity is not a spectator sport. Nurses cannot and should not stand on the sidelines while inequity grows deeper roots. We can be champions of the equity message.

There is no healthcare issue that can truly be considered "someone else's problem." What affects one affects us all. The effects may not be immediate or obvious to all, but in time inequity will cause harm to more than just the groups on the margins. There are many ways for nurses to advocate for equity, and the first step is to recognize it as a critical part of our role and responsibility.

INTRODUCTION

The American Nurses Association (ANA), the American Association of Colleges of Nursing (AACN), the National Academy of Medicine (NAM), the Association for Nursing Professional Development (ANPD), and numerous other organizations have recently highlighted the significant need for diversity, equity, and inclusion in nursing education and practice. While data show increasing diversity within the U.S. population, the nursing profession continues to lag in recruitment and retention of nurses representing the residents of the communities they serve. The above organizations have created executive-level goals and priorities for achieving a more balanced nursing workforce, though there are currently no grassroots initiatives to provide strategies for realistic, attainable, and meaningful change.

Journey to Equity evolved from a conversation in March 2021 between the coeditors who initially planned to develop and publish a white paper on the topic. Over the next several weeks, they discovered that health equity required more than a single paper, and the result was the creation of this book. As the coeditors could not represent the diverse populations impacted by inequities in our population and profession, they sought the input of nurse leaders who represent these communities.

As communities diversify, the nursing profession must rise to the challenge of truly representing the communities they serve. In this book, a historic perspective evolves into a nursing process approach that incorporates the personal stories of nurses with diverse racial, gender, and ethnic backgrounds who share their journeys and their recommendations for the future. This is a template for K–12 schools, community and healthcare organizations, academic and continuing nursing education advocates, and professional associations and organizations to facilitate the growth and success of underrepresented groups in the nursing profession.

Journey to Equity will help readers develop an action plan that meets ANA, AACN, NAM, ANPD, and other initiatives for diversity, inclusion, and equity as nurses lead change and improvement in health care now and into the future.

Beginning the Journey

Carol Susan "Sue" Johnson, PhD, RN,
NE-BC, NPD-BC, FAAN

Why should we be concerned about equity in nursing and health care? What is the impact of equity on social determinants of health and health outcomes? These questions are essential to understanding the context of the *Future of Nursing 2020–2030: Charting a Path to Achieve Health Equity* (National Academies of Science, Engineering, and Medicine [NASEM], 2021). This momentous report can change the U.S. healthcare system by leveraging nurses' contributions to achieve health equity. If the nation is to thrive, everyone must live the healthiest possible life, and helping people achieve this goal is an essential role of nurses in all settings.

However, a diverse nursing workforce must be developed to meet the challenges of inequities in health and health care access in immigrant, rural, and marginalized populations within communities. The stories included here chart the personal and professional journeys of nurse leaders who are representative of racial, ethnic, immigrant, and gender identity groups. Their challenges and successes provide a blueprint for others to seek nursing careers and guide marginalized populations to health equity.

The majority of registered nurses in the United States are White women, despite attempts in recent years to diversify the profession. As the country itself becomes more diverse, nurses must reflect the people and communities they serve to ensure that individuals receive culturally competent care. Equitable health care services must become a reality as we begin the journey to equity. With this in mind, the ANA Enterprise 2020–2023 Strategic Plan established the vision of a healthy world through the power of nursing by evolving the practice of nursing to transform health and health care (American Nurses Association [ANA], 2020). To achieve this goal, ANA is committed to addressing racism in nursing in collaboration with multiple nursing organizations in the National Commission to Address Racism in Nursing, while promoting diversity, equity, and inclusion (ANA, 2021b). Our patients/clients and our profession deserve nothing less.

The Context of the Nursing Profession

How does nursing compare to the population of the United States?
    Two pieces of data are essential to address this question.
Every 2 years, the National Council of State Boards of Nursing (NCSBN) and the National Forum of State Nursing Workforce Centers conduct the only national-level survey about the entire U.S. nursing workforce. Data from 2020 provide valuable information about the diversity of the nursing workforce (Smiley et al., 2021).

Table 1-1. Gender Distribution of Registered Nurses 2020

Gender	N	%
Male	3,915.2	9.4
Female	37,739.9	90.5
Other	43.6	0.1

Male nurses have increased 0.3 percentage points from 2017, and 2020 was the first time the category of "other" could be selected, resulting in selection by 0.1% of nurses. Male nurses also account for 13.6% of all multiracial nurses and 34.3% of nurses identifying as Native Hawaiian or other Pacific Islanders.

Table 1-2. Race of Registered Nurses 2020

Race	N	%
American Indian or Alaska Native	19,391	0.5
Asian	299,340	7.2
Black/African American	279,799	6.7
Native Hawaiian or other Pacific Islander	17,573	0.4
Middle Eastern/North African	8,931	0.2
White/Caucasian	3,356,257	80.6
Other	86,676	2.3
More than one race category selected	88,195	2.1

Nurses who reported being Asian represented the largest non-White/Caucasian racial group in the workforce, although there was a slight decrease (0.3 percentage points) from 2017. The proportion of Black/African American registered nurses increased 0.5 percentage points from 2017. Middle Eastern/North African was a new category in 2020. Nurses reporting being Hispanic/Latinx increased 0.3 percentage points from 2017.

Table 1-3. Hispanic or Latinx Ethnicity of Registered Nurses 2020

Ethnicity	N	%
Hispanic or Latinx	233,364	5.6
Non-Hispanic or Latinx	3,910,949	94.4

It is critical to examine statistics on the nursing workforce in relation to that of the U.S. population, as reflected in the 2020 United States Census Data. Although a final report is not yet available, there is sufficient data to determine changes in racial and ethnic composition of the United States in 2020 (U.S. Census Bureau, 2021a).

Table 1-4. Racial and Ethnic U.S. Census Data 2020

Race/Ethnicity	N (in millions)	%
American Indian or Alaska Native	3.7	1.1
Asian	19.9	6.0
Black/African American	41.1	12.4
Native Hawaiian or other Pacific Islander	0.7	0.2
Hispanic/Latino	62.1	18.7
White/Caucasian	204.3	61.6
Other	27.9	8.4
More than one race category selected	33.8	10.2

Although the White/Caucasian population remained the largest race or ethnicity group in the 2020 census, this population declined by 8.6% since 2010. The Hispanic/Latino population grew 23% in the same time period. The Black or African American population grew 5.6%, and the American Indian and Alaska Native population grew 27.1%. The Asian population grew 35.5% in the years between 2010 and 2020.

Sexual orientation and gender identity were unavailable in the 2020 census data but are currently tracked in the U.S. Census Bureau's Household Pulse Survey. This process began in July 2021, and the following data is from July 27, 2021, to September 13, 2021, for population members aged 18 years and over (U.S. Census Bureau, 2021b).

Table 1-5. U.S. Gender Identity and Sexual Orientation According to the Household Pulse Survey 2021

Gender Identity

Sex assigned on original birth certificate	%	Currently consider self as	%
Female	51.6	Female	50.5
		Transgender	0.6
		Male	0.3
		None of these	1.7
Male	48.4	Male	47.2
		Transgender	0.6
		Female	0.4
		None of these	1.7

Sexual Orientation—Which best represents how you think of yourself?

Sexual orientation	%
Bisexual	4.4
Gay or lesbian	3.3
Straight	83.3
Something else	1.9
I don't know	2.1

Since the racial/ethnic/gender makeup of each community is different, for this data to be useful in building an equitable nursing workforce, it must be examined on a local basis by communities throughout the United States. If the nursing profession is to truly reflect community racial/ethnic/gender composition, emphasis on education for upward mobility must begin during middle and high school years for students in these groups. Visibility of nurses in these settings and at after-school programs for these students (including males) will enhance role modeling and students' awareness about nursing practice and opportunities.

The History of Equity in Nursing Education and Practice

Florence Nightingale is credited as the founder of modern nursing, but nursing has existed since ancient civilizations throughout the world. Religious orders cared for the sick in the Middle Ages, and the Crusaders established and staffed hospitals during the Crusades to control religious sites in the Middle East. The Reformation in England in the 16th century initiated the "Dark Period of Nursing" between 1550 and 1850, when women from the dregs of society, including convicts, were assigned as nurses with no training or experience. Nursing became a women's occupation, and as medicine advanced, nursing remained mired in squalor in hospitals and asylums. The only bright spot was the work of religious orders, like the Sisters of Charity who took charge of hospitals, asylums, and charity work in France. Unfortunately, England's nurses were illiterate, untrained, inconsiderate, and frequently alcoholic. They routinely labored long hours for little pay and supplemented their meager income by taking bribes or stealing from their patients (Donahue, 2011).

Nursing was not an occupation for gentlewomen in the 1850s until Florence Nightingale (1820–1910) determined that nursing was her calling and changed nursing education and practice from then until today (Cook, 1913a, 1913b).

Nursing Education

Although she was well educated for her time, Florence Nightingale's formal nursing education consisted of 2 weeks of observation in 1850 at Kaiserswerth Institute in Germany and one month of rudimentary training there in 1851. In February of 1853, she went to Paris, where she observed hospitals and nurses, but family matters required her to return home without enrolling in an apprenticeship program (Cook, 1913a). Her subsequent service in the Crimean War resulted in the establishment of the Nightingale Fund by the British people to recognize the contribution of Nightingale and her nurses. In 1861, this fund supported the first nurses' training program—the Nightingale Training School at St. Thomas's Hospital in London (Dossey et al., 2005). The Nightingale School served as a template for other nurse training programs both in England and the United States.

There were no nursing schools in the United States until the New England Hospital for Women and Children in Boston started one in 1872. The first applicant, Linda Richards, graduated a year later as the first trained American nurse. Her education consisted of lectures by physicians on medicine, surgery, and obstetrics. Clinical work from 0530 to 2100 required the five students to care for six patients each. Students learned from female interns how to take vital signs and provide physical care. There were no textbooks and no entrance or final exams. Richards wasn't satisfied with her own knowledge and skills. She eventually became superintendent of the nurse training school at Massachusetts General Hospital and convinced the trustees that she should spend time in England gaining experience at their training schools. In May 1877, Linda Richards met Florence Nightingale and was able to spend time at St. Thomas's Hospital, King's College Hospital, the Royal Infirmary, and hospitals in Paris with Nightingale's blessing. Richards held numerous leadership positions in her career due to the knowledge she acquired beyond her basic nursing education (Richards, 1911).

Richards's experience in nursing education mirrored many of her contemporaries. During the rest of the 19th and 20th centuries, nursing education gradually progressed from total subservience and servitude to classwork, textbooks, and examinations for proficiency. Nurse leaders in education such as Isabel Hampton Robb, Adelaide Nutting, Annie Goodrich, Elizabeth Carnegie, and Virginia Henderson advanced nursing education toward professional status (Johnson, 2016). Over time, many diploma schools gave way to associate degree and baccalaureate nursing programs, and nurses pursued master's and doctoral education to elevate the profession.

Diversity in Early Days of Nursing in the U.S.

Nightingale focused her school on White women, and most American training schools did the same. The first African American trained nurse was Mary Eliza Mahoney, who enrolled in 1878 in the training program at the New England Hospital for Women and Children. Her experience was similar to that of Linda Richards, working 16-hour days on wards with responsibility for six patients. During the 16-month course, the majority of students dropped out and Mahoney was one of only four graduates from a class of 42 (Johnson, 2016). Her career will be profiled under the nursing practice section.

Elizabeth Carnegie attended the Lincoln School for Nurses in New York City after graduating from an African American high school in Washington, D.C. The students were Black, but the director and all instructors were White. Ms. Carnegie subsequently received a bachelor's degree in sociology from West Virginia State College (an African American school). As her career advanced, she obtained a fellowship from the Rockefeller Foundation to obtain a certificate in nursing school administration at the University of Toronto. A second fellowship enabled Carnegie to obtain a master's of education from Syracuse University. She became dean of the Florida A&M Nursing Program for African American Nurses and overcame prejudice to gain clinical experiences for her students, procure student housing, and raise academic standards (Johnson, 2016).

Estelle Massey Riddle Osborne demonstrated an ability to move freely in both segregated and integrated groups. Seizing every opportunity for professional development, she became the first African American nurse with a master's degree in nursing education. However, her greatest impact on nursing education was increasing the number of nursing schools accepting African American women and improving access to higher education for African American nurses (Johnson, 2016).

Luther Christman became a nurse when it wasn't an accepted career for men. After education roles at the University of Michigan and Vanderbilt, where he was the first man to be nursing dean, he accepted a position at Rush University in Chicago to develop nursing programs there. Although Mr. Christman experienced prejudice against men in nursing during his career, he was instrumental in establishing the Rush Model, a unified approach to nursing education, research, and practice. Another major accomplishment of his was implementing nurse practitioner and clinical doctoral programs when few clinical degrees were available (Johnson, 2016).

Nursing Practice

Nightingale's first nursing position as superintendent of the Hospital for Gentlewomen During Illness at Harley Street in London enabled her to participate in patient care, supervise nurses, coordinate construction, facilitate patient discharges, reduce operating costs, and use political savvy in reporting to two committees in charge: the Committee of Ladies and the Committee of Gentleman (responsible for finances). Her experience at Harley Street prepared her for managing nurses in a war zone less than a year later.

Nightingale continued to serve as a role model in care delivery and formed alliances with some physicians, orderlies, and influential officials to advance cleanliness and safety. She deferred to physicians in medical matters and ensured that she and her nurses complied with rules and regulations (Cook, 1913a). Later in her life, she admonished nurses to focus on direct patient care (e.g., cleanliness, positioning, feeding, bandaging, bed making, cooking) and was concerned about their punctuality, quietness, trustworthiness, personal neatness and cleanliness, and ability to manage a ward (Dossey et al., 2005). Her major contribution to the nursing process was her emphasis on careful observation so nurses could accurately report patient changes to physicians, and her focus on well care continues today. She considered nursing a calling, not a profession (Cook, 1913a; Cook, 1913b).

This focus on tasks continued in nursing practice in both England and the United States until the late 1950s when Ida Jean Orlando's Nursing Process Theory (assessment, diagnosis, planning, implementation, and evaluation) created a framework for patient-centered care that considered nursing as a distinct profession separate from medicine. In her theory, nurses determine nursing actions beyond physician orders and involve patients in their care process (Current Nursing, 2020).

In the years since then, nursing roles have expanded from the bedside to the boardroom. Nurses today use their skills in multiple settings and as valued members of interprofessional teams.

Impact of Diversity in Nursing Practice

Minority nurses have impacted clinical practice since the 1870s. Since hospitals did not employ staff nurses in the United States, Mary Eliza Mahoney, the first African American trained nurse, joined the Nurses Directory after graduation and did private duty nursing for about 30 years. Her patients loved her, and her expertise and professionalism made her a role model for equal opportunity for African American women (Johnson, 2016).

Susie Walking Bear Yellowtail became the first Apsáalooke (Crow) registered nurse in the United States in 1923. When working at the Bureau of Indian Affairs Hospital on the reservation (1929–1931) she encountered blatant discrimination toward Native Americans, with women being sterilized without their consent. Her outrage led to a role as healthcare advocate, representing the U.S. Public Health Service in assessing and providing midwifery care for women in the Little Horn Valley for 30 years. She joined state health advisory boards and eventually became the spokeswoman for Native Americans on reservations, advocating for expanded access to care, better health care, and improved living conditions (Johnson, 2016).

Mabel Keaton Staupers began her nursing career as a private duty nurse but became active in tuberculosis-related issues in New York City in the 1920s. She organized lectures on health education for the public, established fresh-air summer camps for children, and developed health services that included free examinations and dental care for school children. She also created prenatal clinics and advocated for the appointment of African American physicians to TB clinics and hospitals in New York City. Her focus on advocacy made her a national figure in the fight for equality and integration in nursing in the United States (Johnson, 2016).

Henrieta Villaescusa became the only Hispanic Public Health Supervisor in the L.A. Health Department and embarked on a career of public service in state, national, and international arenas. She was a pioneer in addressing the needs of Hispanic people with diabetes and established innovative, nationwide community participation programs for the Office of Health Affairs. As a member of the Alliance for Progress in the 1960s, Villaescusa helped improve Latin American health by enlisting community and academic nurse leaders to collaborate with local health professionals in Bolivia, Ecuador, Panama, and Peru. As a member of the Task Force on Minority Health, she represented the health needs of Hispanic people in the United States (National Association of Hispanic Nurses, 2021; Legacy.com, 2005).

Current Focus on Diversity in Nursing

In 2021, the American Nurses Association stated the importance of lifelong learning in *Nursing: Scope and Standards of Practice (4th Edition)* within a new standard called Respectful and Equitable Practice which included this statement as a registered nurse competency: "Participates in life-long learning to understand cultural preferences, worldviews, choices, and decision-making processes of diverse consumers" (ANA, 2021c, p. 93).

In 2022, the Association for Nursing Professional Development's updated *Nursing Professional Development: Scope and Standards of Practice* also includes a new standard related to respectful and equitable practice (Harper & Maloney, 2022). This standard provides a guide for Nursing Professional Development (NPD) practitioners to use in collaboration with organizational leadership and community groups in their role as allies to marginalized group members. Cultural humility is an attribute that NPD practitioners integrate in their personal and professional growth as they focus on diversity, inclusion, and equity in educational, recruitment, and retention strategies. As NPD practitioners increase their self-awareness and reflect critically on assumptions and potential biases, they identify and implement strategies to eliminate unfavorable stereotypes and biases. They role-model culturally sensitive and humble behaviors, and their own development and growth enables them to guide the journey to equity in both the organization and community (Harper & Maloney, 2022).

Opportunities to Improve Equity in Nursing
Nurse Academic Faculty: The Beginning of Equity

Nursing academic faculty play a pivotal role in preparing students of diverse backgrounds to care for an increasingly diverse population. Currently, these faculty are primarily White women who do not reflect the makeup of their students or the population they will serve. As nurse educators retire, there is a shortage of available faculty members that is impacting the ability to admit students who are representative of their communities (NASEM, 2021). Several of our authors described a feeling of isolation in their nursing education programs, and some sought mentors within their culture to help them navigate their academic experience. Having more faculty members who are representative of their community can make the transition to nursing easier and more effective for students who otherwise will struggle to enter the profession.

Accrediting bodies establish minimum standards for nursing education programs to prepare graduates for the licensing examination (NCLEX). The majority of clinical experiences have been in acute care settings, but there is a need for nurses to address social determinants of health (SDOH), and these experiences are found in community settings where diverse populations experience poverty, food insecurity, and limited access to health services. Many of these individuals have two or more comorbidities, requiring ongoing monitoring and treatment modalities. Students from minority backgrounds bring personal experience with SDOH's impact on communities to their education program and can share insight into how to gain the trust of these individuals.

In 2019, the National League for Nursing (NLN) published the *Vision for Integration of the Social Determinants of Health Into Nursing Education Curricula* (NLN, 2019). This document relates SDOH to nursing's mission and recommends how to integrate SDOH into nursing education programs. In 2021, the American Association of Colleges of Nursing (AACN) published *The Essentials: Core Competencies for Professional Nursing Education* with curriculum content and expected competencies for graduates of nursing programs (AACN, 2021). Baccalaureate education should emphasize population health, health equity, and SDOH. Unfortunately, these concepts are not well integrated into nursing education at the undergraduate and graduate levels. The Committee on the Future of Nursing 2020–2030 found a lack of analysis and systematic study of these programs and that these recommendations have not yet become standard practice across nursing curriculums (NASEM, 2021). This committee found that most programs use public health or community nursing courses to include content on SDOH in underserved, vulnerable populations. However, a single course offering does not integrate this content into the entire curriculum and is not enough to prepare graduates to address SDOH. Integration is essential for students to adequately understand how social determinants contribute to health inequities. Lack of experiential and community-based learning limits competency development for future practice.

Although further research is recommended, it is time for nursing programs to thoroughly integrate SDOH in curricula and have faculty who are diverse and able to relate to their students and the community itself. These faculty members must ensure that curricula support SDOH, nursing's social mission, and health equity. This includes partnerships with community agencies to provide experiences about the impact of SDOH on individuals, at-risk populations, and community members in varied clinical settings. Their expertise must provide students with new perspectives about how social determinants impact population differences and how to mitigate bias and racism. Not all current faculty members are adept in this new approach to nursing education. This, combined with faculty retirements and vacancies, adversely influences the ability of nursing education programs to pivot to this new approach.

Faculty recruitment and education about implicit and explicit bias, inclusivity, health and wellness initiatives, addressing racism, health equity, and linkage to nursing's social mission is essential if programs are to succeed in the next decade. This will not be an easy transition, but a necessary one (NASEM, 2021).

Nurse Leaders: Mitigating Bias and Racism

Nurse leaders from unit managers to chief nursing officers (CNOs) are responsible for the functioning and teamwork of their nursing and interprofessional colleagues. They must understand the role of culture in xenophobia, ethnocentrism, prejudice, and racism. Culture has been defined in various ways but is inclusive of people who share interests, beliefs, and perspectives. While this identification with a specific group is not necessarily negative, it can result in intolerance toward other groups who do not fit these preconceptions. In extreme cases, this can result in xenophobia or ethnocentrism. Baldwin (2017) defines relevant terms: *xenophobia* refers to fear, mistrust, or dislike of groups or people seen as different from the in-group; *ethnocentrism* complements this by seeing the dominant culture as superior to others; *prejudice* is a negative consequence of such beliefs and actions. Prejudice favors one group over another based on thoughts, behaviors, rhetoric, and policies. *Racism* is a type of prejudice where intolerance is based on race, ethnicity, gender, and sexual orientation. This exists in individuals and society and results in exclusion in communication, policies, and laws.

Everyone is biased based on past experiences that shape their perspectives. Explicit biases are attitudes and beliefs people consciously have about others if they perceive them to be a threat. Focusing on common aspects between individuals and groups can diffuse these biases. Implicit biases are difficult to resolve because they may be unconscious, and people are unaware of them (Falker, 2021).

With this framework, nurse leaders can begin to mitigate racism and bias in the work environment for themselves and others. The first step is to recognize awareness of their own biases by consciously examining negative thoughts and why they exist. This is not an easy process, but nurse leaders must be role models for others by checking their own biases and working to overcome them (Falker, 2021).

All nurse leaders must ensure that education of themselves and others is the first step on this journey. However, a single education session is not enough. If bias and racism are to be mitigated in clinical practice, everyone must walk the walk. Knowledge must be followed by skills and practice for attitudes to truly change. Bringing groups together in open forums and projects will provide opportunities to dispel negative perceptions about others by increasing collaboration and communication.

Nurse leaders can encourage celebrations for community populations where staff members of those groups can share cultural information with others. They also need to determine if communications, procedures, policies, and strategic plans are nondiscriminatory. Nurse leaders must use their voices to promote diversity, inclusion, and equity through their daily awareness and work to address social inequities with the interprofessional team and at structural and policy levels (Baldwin, 2017). They have a unique opportunity to collaborate with other departments, such as human resources, quality management, finance, and the executive team, to ensure that policies and procedures reflect inclusion and equity.

Community Nurses and Professional Connections: Equity and Social Determinants of Health

Community nurses serve in a variety of roles that include public health, community clinics, home care agencies, rural health care, prison/jail nurses, and school nurses. Each role is unique and complementary in addressing equity and social determinants of health. Health equity is essential for everyone to lead a healthier life but often is not achievable for disadvantaged, low-income, and rural communities as well as people of color. There are multiple reasons for this inequity that are tied to social determinants of health, including economic stability, education, social and community context, health and health care, neighborhood, and environmental influences such as food access, crime, and housing. (NASEM, 2021).

How can community nurses assess the populations they serve for SDOH and equity? The answer is different depending on the nurse's role and community clients. The nurse must be able to relate to individuals based on their unique needs. This can be difficult without shared experiences, but nurses must use their knowledge and expertise to understand their client's needs and concerns.

Economic stability can be assessed in interviews or a nursing history. Is the individual employed in a job that meets their needs, or are they unemployed or underemployed? Inadequate income exacerbates poverty and housing instability. The individual may be choosing between food or medicine and a place to stay. This is not just an urban issue. It also impacts rural populations. Nurses in home care, public health, and community clinics must focus on economic stability in assessing clients' needs. This also impacts school nurses who see children who are homeless and come to school hungry and too tired to study in class. Careful assessment is key to providing support that meets these children's needs (NASEM, 2021).

Education is vital to reduce poverty and enable individuals to seek employment opportunities that will increase income. Members of at-risk populations often lack educational opportunities, from early childhood education and development to high school graduation. For these individuals, enrollment in higher education is unattainable. School nurses have an opportunity to talk with teachers and school social workers to determine at-risk children who struggle in school and consider dropping out. The nurse's assessment can assist with a plan to help the student succeed. Some of the nurses who share their stories in this book were supported to get a high school degree or GED and move on to nursing programs. Counselors, teachers, and nurses can play a key role in students' future success.

Literacy is another aspect that must be addressed. Nurses in community clinics and public health have a responsibility to assess reading literacy of both children and adults and connect them to resources that will prepare them for future education and better employment (NASEM, 2021).

Social and community context is important for individuals and populations to improve health equity. Poor quality, unsafe neighborhoods can limit healthcare resources available to residents in urban and rural settings. Community nurses can screen clients in relation to social factors and refer them to appropriate community resources for support. They can also advocate for a community's residents by supporting laws and regulations that will improve health for all people. Nurses who work with incarcerated individuals can assess what they will need to succeed on the outside as responsible members of society. These nurses can then collaborate with officials and social services to provide inmates with educational and social resources. Nurses in all community settings can promote social cohesion to move neighborhoods toward health equity (NASEM, 2021).

Health and health care include access issues and health literacy. Access to primary care is essential for positive health outcomes and prevents illness and death. Unfortunately, lack of insurance reduces preventive care and care for chronic diseases and major health conditions. Health literacy impacts health equity in at-risk populations who cannot obtain, process, and/or understand basic health information to make appropriate health decisions. Community nurses must carefully assess clients' understanding and ability to use health information to begin increasing health literacy (NASEM, 2021).

Neighborhood and environmental influences encompass a wide variety of factors, including access to healthy foods, incidence of violence and crime, environmental conditions, and housing quality. Community nurses must assess the environment of the population they serve by asking the following questions: Is there access to healthy food in the area? What is the crime rate? Do residents feel safe? Are there environmental hazards? Is housing inadequate? These answers will enable community nurses in public health, community clinics, home care agencies, rural health care, prison/jail settings, and schools to assess the current situation and plan to address the SDOH and move toward health equity (NASEM, 2021).

Building professional connections is an essential skill for all nurses in community settings. Since it is impossible to address all these issues singlehandedly, an interprofessional approach involving teachers, school counselors, mental health professionals, substance use specialists, legal advocates, and community activists will enable community nurses to assist others on the journey to health equity and improving the social determinants of health.

Advanced Practice Registered Nurses: Equity and Person-Centered Care

Advanced practice registered nurses (APRNs) have a master's degree or higher in nursing and can improve health equity by focusing on patient-centered care. However, their ability to achieve positive results is adversely impacted in multiple areas where practice restrictions exist. In 2011, the Institute of Medicine report *The Future of Nursing: Leading Change, Advancing Health* made four recommendations related to advanced practice nurses: (1) nurses should practice to the full extent of their training and education; (2) nurses should obtain higher levels of training and education through seamless academic progression; (3) nurses should be full partners with other healthcare colleagues, including physicians, to redesign health care in the U.S.; and (4) effective policymaking and workforce planning require improved data collection and infrastructure for information (IOM, 2011).

Although some progress has been made in the past decade, 27 states do not allow full practice authority for advanced practice nurses. Nurse practitioners (NPs) in these states cannot prescribe medication, diagnose patients, or provide treatment without an agreement with a physician. In 11 states, physician oversight is required for all practice by NPs. The National Academies have reiterated this recommendation in their new publication because advanced practice nurses are integral to improve access to quality care and health equity (NASEM, 2021).

APRNs can diagnose and treat illnesses or health conditions, advise members of the public on health issues, manage chronic diseases, and provide preventive care services while engaging in continuous professional development to stay abreast of methodological, technological, and other developments in their specialties. Their focus on person-centered care and their ability as advocates for health equity can improve social determinants of health outcomes for individuals, communities, and at-risk populations when they can practice at the top of their license and education (NASEM, 2021).

Nurse Researchers/Scientists: Addressing Health Equity

Nurse researchers/scientists have a significant role to play in the journey to health equity. A sound evidence base is needed to determine the impact of nursing interventions on SDOH, health equity, environmental health, and population health. Nurse researchers/ scientists need to design and conduct studies that will identify and integrate examples of SDOH—economic stability, education, health and health care, social and community context, and neighborhood and environmental factors—to improve nursing care coordination for individuals, families, and community populations. Their results will also impact how community nurse administrators and human resource departments focus on recruiting and retaining nurses who reflect the communities they serve (NASEM, 2021).

This is new research territory for many nurse researchers/scientists, and comprehensive education must be provided about SDOH, population health, and health equity to develop their expertise. The National Institute of Nursing Research is an excellent resource to prepare them to address these research gaps (NASEM, 2021). As information technology advances, nurse researchers/scientists can use artificial intelligence and virtual services to address SDOH and health equity. There will be opportunities to explore how nurses' roles impact health equity and health disparities. Knowledge of disadvantaged groups will enable nurse researchers to determine if interventions reduce disparities within these groups and how this occurs. There is also a need for longitudinal studies about nurse-led/nurse-involved health equity interventions and their effectiveness and sustainability over time (NASEM, 2021).

Nurse researchers/scientists must also use the expertise they have gained in population health to partner with key community stakeholders in designing research studies that are applicable to the population. New health models must be explored to see if they meet individual and population needs. Related public and organizational policies at public health, community, and health system levels must be investigated to ensure that they improve health and health equity (NASEM, 2021).

There is also a need to recruit and retain nurses who mirror the diverse, ethnic, and cultural backgrounds of community populations. This must be a priority for nurse researchers/scientists who will investigate whether innovative approaches in K–12 STEM education and mentoring/support that give underrepresented students opportunities for classroom success are effective nursing recruitment avenues. Much of this research will consist of longitudinal studies and may also include summer pipeline programs and focused high school healthcare education that provides high school and college credits simultaneously. If nurse researchers/scientists' study results demonstrate the effectiveness of such approaches, this evidence can be used to reduce barriers in the pathway from high school to recruitment, admission, retention, and academic success in nursing programs to licensure and advancement in nursing (NASEM, 2021).

This is a call to action for nurse researchers/scientists and a significant research agenda. It will take knowledge, time, skills, and dedication, but the results of reducing health disparities, advancing health equity, and recruiting and retaining nurses who reflect the communities they serve—make it worthwhile.

Acute Care Nurses and the Interprofessional Team: Equity in Practice

Addressing equity in practice is not solely the responsibility of nurses in acute care settings. It requires a team approach where all participants collaborate to reduce racism and bias and advance toward equity in practice. Acute care nurses must begin by understanding and valuing the contributions of each interprofessional team member. Each member brings knowledge and skills that are essential for all patients to receive equitable health care. The team can include nursing, medicine, allied health professionals (e.g., dietitians, physical therapists, respiratory therapists, occupational therapists, social workers), and other departments (e.g., quality, infection prevention, risk management; Kaini, 2017).

Team members must pool their skills, knowledge, and expertise to develop and achieve mutually agreed-upon goals that will provide optimal desired outcomes and patient satisfaction. This is a dynamic process where the team collaborates to benefit and empower the patient and family by complementing each other in their professional roles. The nurse is a major player who realizes that effective communication by team members must promote team collaboration, problem solving, and decision making. Actual leadership roles will change based on specific care situations. Respect for others' capabilities and contributions is essential for interprofessional team success (Kaini, 2017).

In the context of equity, the nurse must be alert to personal and professional structural racism and bias. Patients are diverse, from different ethnic and cultural groups, and many suffer from health inequity gaps that may adversely impact their health care. Negative stereotypes and beliefs can create implicit biases and racism that are detrimental to developing a caring relationship with patients who don't fit with providers' perceptions. Nurses must be alert to discrimination toward these patients and confront it in themselves and others. Reflecting on their own biases and getting to know patients and their care goals is essential to move beyond stereotypes and really see the individuals beyond the diagnosis (NASEM, 2021).

Just dealing with their own biases and racism is not enough for nurses on interprofessional teams. As part of team leadership, nurses must set an example of inclusion and address negative and toxic cultural norms by other team members, including the nursing staff in the acute care setting. Interprofessional teams have an opportunity to learn from each other and teach each other. The acute care nurse plays an integral role in helping the interprofessional team put equity into practice to improve patient outcomes and satisfaction (Kaini, 2017; NASEM, 2021).

A Nursing Process Approach to Achieving Equity Assessment

For the journey to equity in nursing to be successful, the process must begin by identifying racial and ethnic groups in the community and understanding how they view health care, education, and their social determinants of health. Gender assessment must also be considered to understand how male and transgender individuals view these considerations.

Equity in assessment does not mean identical experiences, just that assessment practice and interpretation of results are fair and just for all groups. Although equality of outcome is not possible, equality of access is the goal. This assessment can result in curriculum and/or practice changes that promote access by marginalized groups.

Assessment for equity involves collecting and analyzing information via multiple data-gathering processes to determine the extent to which a program or other resource is equitable to each community member. This provides opportunities to deeply examine all aspects of an academic institution to uncover institutional strengths and weaknesses related to equity (Equity Literacy Institute, 2021).

According to the Equity Literacy Institute, these assessments can be broad to incorporate a wide variety of formal reports and data gathering. It can also be more limited in scope and focus on individual initiatives or programs. Nurses and other assessment team members must collaborate to create focus group protocols, surveys, and data collection instruments to reflect unique opportunities and challenges in the specific context. Assessment instruments must be relevant and accessible to multiple constituencies. The team helps organizations explore a broad range of equity issues and where they intersect. This includes gender identity, race, socioeconomic status, sexual orientation, religion, language, (dis)ability, and immigrant status. Assessment teams use a variety of qualitative and quantitative methods for data collection and focus beyond just completing the assessment to preparing organizations to develop an ongoing assessment process. Constituencies/stakeholders must be interpreted broadly so no essential data is missed (Equity Literacy Institute, 2021).

Planning

The American Planning Association (APA) ratified a *Planning for Equity Policy Guide* in 2019 (Ross et al., 2019) to promote equity and remove barriers in policies and regulations that prolong inequity in the United States. This document provides a clear framework to advance principles of sound planning by including all community members in planning equity. Planners must understand demographic changes related to age, gender, ethnicity, cultural and religious backgrounds, and other characteristics impacting planning within the United States. It is imperative that planners behave ethically to ensure social equity as they develop policies. APA membership now includes 45% women and 15% minorities, but this diversification must continue to reflect the communities served. The planning pillars of diversity, inclusion, and equity are guides for planners as they seek to make all communities great for everyone. Nurses can be key players in engagement with assessment and planning teams.

Since planners deal with policy issues, specific policies are essential for community engagement and empowerment. Everyone must have a voice and access to informed decision-making. Frequently, distribution of community resources is strongly influenced by single-family homeowners who are mainly White and above median income. Projects that would benefit disadvantaged, lower income community members are often unheard or denied. Planners must ensure that there is meaningful participation and outreach to all populations. This includes renters, lower income households, people of color, youth, the elderly, families, and homeless community members.

Nurses in community settings can foster community engagement by reaching out to engage marginalized members, those with disabilities, language barriers, literacy issues, and unavailability due to work and family responsibilities. They may use interpreters, incorporate devices for people with hearing impairments, review materials for an acceptable reading level, and ensure translation of materials as needed for comprehension. Nurses who are part of these planning teams must ensure that community members have a meaningful voice in outcomes and decisions as well as ensuring that these contributions are documented and addressed. Open communication and active listening are essential to create trust, develop deliverable outcomes, and follow through on actions that prioritize the goals of local residents and partners, particularly those of marginalized populations (Ross et al., 2019).

Another aspect of the APA planning process deals with health equity, essential for those considering a nursing career (Ross et al., 2019). Achieving health equity requires improved healthcare access, promotion of health impact assessments, and implementation of health equity policies. Health Impact Assessments can be used to focus on equity and sustainability in health issues. Health equity policies focus on improving the quality of living and community health through planning with an equity focus (Ross et al., 2019).

Health equity must include all involved parties—planners, community members, public health departments, healthcare professionals, and community organizations. Multiple perspectives are essential to completely understand and address health inequities. Education about social determinants of health is integral to apply equity principles in community planning. Planning is not a short-term process. Long-range community needs for access to services, fresh foods, and environmental planning must not be overlooked. Healthcare access may mean better public transportation and use of treatment/education centers in underserved areas, such as community centers, schools, senior centers, and other non-traditional settings. (Ross et al., 2019).

Implementation

Equity must be at the center of implementation. The Annie E. Casey Foundation, the National Implementation Network, and the William T. Grant Foundation collaborated to develop a concept of equitable implementation as a blueprint for success (Woo et al., 2019). Equitable implementation integrates the tools and principles of implementation science with equity components, including specific attention to the values, culture, history, and needs of the community. Effective community programs require equity for knowledge development and use. This means implementation must change to achieve equitable outcomes.

Nurses and other planners must ensure equity in those who create a practice, those who use and validate the practice, and those who are impacted by the practice. They must create teams that distribute responsibility, accountability, and power while embracing flexibility and complexity instead of a single right answer or approach. Cultural knowledge and expertise must be incorporated in the implementation process.

There are several examples of how various groups can use equitable implementation in practice. These groups may include community members, funders, researchers, and practitioners who interact in the following ways: *Community members* are integral players in implementation from beginning to end—from need definition, assessing, choosing, and implementing interventions, providing data, input, and interpretation of findings that may change implementation priorities. *Funders* are patient to await outcomes and realize the difference between equitable outcomes for all and improved outcomes for some. They are partners who promote equal voice and power, not as a privileged funder. *Researchers* are open to community experiences and realize how their assumptions impact their work. They identify the core and adaptable components of the developed and validated intervention and provide technical support that considers and reflects cultural norms. They also serve as co-learners in the implementation process and value different ways of knowing. *Practitioners*, including nurses, are open to community experiences and engage community members. They also realize how their assumptions impact their work. They ask what data are needed to determine if an intervention is working and develop capacity to use and critically appraise research by considering how the knowledge base is relevant to the community and how to implement it to promote equity.

Implementation requires that equity clearly addresses disparities. Implementation science must use approaches like those described above to advance equity in communities (Woo et al., 2019).

Evaluation

The current evaluation paradigm focuses on bias, validity, reliability, rigor, and objectivity that seeks generalizable and scaled data and findings that often are not reflective of the community in terms of inequality, equity, or social justice. The Equitable Evaluation Initiative (2020) seeks to change this paradigm to an equitable evaluation format. This may be accomplished by acknowledging that current evaluation conceals racism and privilege as objectivity, exploring how current practices can be barriers to adopting equitable evaluation principles, and identifying and sharing approaches to interrupt these barriers. Evaluative thinking must link organizational strategy, culture, and evaluation as both a leadership competency and organizational capacity. Context and culture must be addressed with definitions that reflect the time, place, and intentions, and the pool of evaluators must be diversified and expanded with new and different ways to understand knowledge, evidence, and truth for greater validity and rigor.

Equitable evaluation principles frame how evaluations should be conducted related to equity. The core of evaluation is the responsibility to advance progress toward equity. The work of nurses and others in evaluation should be culturally valid and focused on participant ownership. Evaluative work should address critical questions such as how historical and structural decisions contributed to the condition being addressed, the effect on strategy of systemic drivers of inequity, and how the cultural context occurs in the structural conditions and change initiative itself (Equitable Evaluation Initiative, 2020).

Foundations, nonprofits, and evaluators must conduct evaluation processes in alignment with these equitable evaluation principles. If not, there is a risk of exacerbating or reinforcing the inequities that the change seeks to resolve (Equitable Evaluation Initiative, 2020).

Use of the nursing process steps—assessment, planning, implementation, and evaluation—can impact opportunities to improve equity of marginalized and underserved community populations when nurses collaborate with other team members to seek viable community-based solutions. As noted in the Future of Nursing report, "To achieve health equity, the committee envisions a major role for the nursing profession in engaging in the complex work of aligning public health, health care, social services, and public policies to eliminate health disparities and achieve health equity" (NASEM, 2021, p. 18).

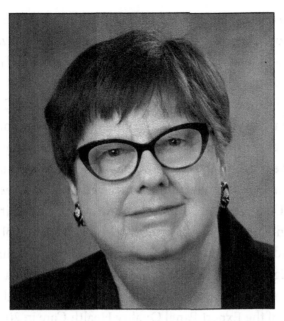

Sue Johnson, PhD, RN, NE-BC, NPD-BE, FAAN
Founder & Principal RN Innovations LLC

Dr. Johnson has been a practicing nurse for over 50 years serving in a variety of healthcare roles, including staff nurse, manager, nursing resource management specialist, accreditation specialist, and director of clinical excellence and nursing research at a Midwest health system. As principal of a company specializing in leadership and professional development education, she advocates for innovation and improvements in health care, especially interprofessional education/collaboration and measurement of nursing economic impact. Dr. Johnson is the author of four books relating Nightingale's vision to advance health through nursing to today's healthcare environment with implications for future practice. Her books, publications, and presentations promote interprofessional education/collaboration in the clinical learning environment and measure how nursing economic impact improves organizational outcomes and quality patient care. Her role as a national nursing and healthcare leader is unique, and she currently serves as vice chair of the Commission on Accreditation for Nursing Continuing Professional Development, on the Nurse Leader Board of AARP, and as a peer reviewer for the *Journal for Nursing Professional Development*. She is a former director of the Association for Nursing Professional Development and has received numerous awards, including Distinguished Alumnus Jamestown Community College, the Golden Hoosier Award by the State of Indiana for volunteer service, and the Lifetime Achievement Award from Xi Nu-at Large Chapter Sigma Theta Tau. Dr. Johnson was inducted as a fellow in the American Academy of Nursing in 2019 and served as vice chair elect of the Expert Panel Quality Health Care in 2021. Dr. Johnson considers this book the most significant achievement of her career and an opportunity to truly achieve equity in the nursing profession.

2

Overcoming Adversity: A Journey to Becoming a Nurse Leader and Entrepreneur

Larissa Africa, MBA, BSN, RN, FAAN

Nursing Runs Through My Veins

"I was born to be a nurse! I had all the Cherry Ames books when I was young," said a nurse during a team building exercise. I smiled, nodded, and thought to myself, "Who is Cherry Ames? I don't know Cherry Ames! Should I know Cherry Ames?" I was in a little bit of a panic. How can I be an effective nurse leader if I don't know Cherry Ames?

Unlike many, I don't have a family full of nurses who forged the path for me. I had one. The first person who introduced me to nursing was my aunt, who after working 2 years as a labor and delivery nurse became a stay-at-home mother but remained the family nurse. At a very young age in the Philippines, I remember watching my aunt care for my ailing grandfather. I was amazed at how she used the sphygmomanometer. What was she listening to? How did she get those numbers she said out loud to a group of us watching just by placing her stethoscope on my grandfather's arm and pumping the black rubber bulb? But, as amazed as I was, I did not have any desire to be a nurse. Nursing was (and still is, in some circles) not seen as a highly regarded profession in the Philippines—nurses are doctor's assistants. They just follow orders. I had no desire to just follow orders. I decided then that I would become a doctor.

I was 12 years old when I immigrated to the United States along with my father, mother, and younger sister. We had what I would call a typical Filipinx immigrant experience. We stayed with relatives for several months, all four of us sharing a 10 × 10 bedroom. My parents slept on one full-sized bed while my sister and I shared the other.

Thankfully, my Catholic school education in the Philippines had prepared me to speak, read, and write in formal "American" English. However, I did not understand some of the slang words that other kids my age were using, which made the transition a difficult one for me. At 12, I was just beginning to figure out who I was. At 12, I had to quickly figure out how to survive in a world I knew nothing about. Food fights in the school cafeteria, kids who could barely read, teachers called by their last names minus the "Mr." or "Ms." were all new experiences. There were times when kids called me "chink" and babbled words that to them were what the Chinese language sounded like. As a new Filipinx immigrant, I was confused and hurt by these comments. Before coming to America, I thought that all of America was like *Dallas*, the soap opera. I had no idea that California is a hub for multiculturalism where people from all over the world would come and soak up the sun and hope for a piece of the American dream. Many spoke a language I did not understand. Most did not look like me. When we moved to a two-bedroom apartment in a mostly Asian community 6 months later, I felt a little bit of relief. I chose to stay at the same junior high school I started in. My mom would wake up early to take a 30-minute bus ride to drop me off at school, and then she would take another 30-minute bus ride home to prepare my sister for school before she went to work herself. My mother had completed her degree in pharmacy but was still a few credits short of being able to sit for the pharmacy exam. She chose not to pursue completing her missing credits and settled for a pharmacy technician job 3 months after our arrival. My father, who has a degree in business administration, found a job in the same hospital 6 months later as a cafeteria worker. Money was always tight. We only bought new outfits for Easter, Christmas, and a few for starting a new school year. We ate home-cooked meals, not because they were a healthier choice but because they were the cheaper choice. Eating a burger at McDonald's was a treat.

My parents made many friends along the way, mostly nurses who worked in the same hospital as they did. We spent many holidays with our fellow Filipinx immigrants—mostly nurses. Some were with their families, some had to leave their spouses and children in the Philippines, and some were with their spouses but the children were left in the care of grandparents. I watched them work 12-hour shifts day in and day out. Some were working two to three jobs to send money back home. They shared stories of their difficult days and how much their feet hurt from standing all day. (Come to think of it, I never heard the good things that happened to them.) I learned about the migration of Filipinx nurses to the United States from stories they told during get-togethers. I heard of doctors in the Philippines becoming nurses here in the United States. I was immersed in the world of nursing at an early age, but still, I didn't want to be a nurse like many Filipinx immigrants.

As high school graduation was coming near, I had to decide what I was going to do with my life. I had no idea what options I had for colleges and universities. UCLA, USC, Harvey-Mudd, NYU, Cal Tech, Penn State—my head was spinning. All I knew was that I wanted a different path for myself than what I had been exposed to for the last 4 years of my life. I wanted options. I wanted stability. I wanted financial security. Frankly, I wanted to be able to afford take-out food because I did not like to cook! For months, I struggled with finding my path. I went over in my head different college degrees, and nothing seemed right. Then after a gathering with family friends, I thought to myself, why not nursing? I'm already surrounded by nurses anyway. They make good money. It's a stable profession. Yes, it's physically demanding, but I can do it. Why not? I volunteered at the hospital where my parents were working. During my first few weeks, I was introduced to different team members. I met the infection control nurse. I met a nurse manager. I met a nurse educator. I met the CNO. Wow! Wait . . . this was not the nursing profession I grew up knowing. There were so many options! I never imagined that nursing could provide so many opportunities. I was excited to tell my parents that I wanted to become a nurse. They were excited for me because they knew how much their nurse friends were making. I remember my parents saying, "You can go to the community college, get your associate degree, and make a lot of money. It would only take you 2 years. You can work for several hospitals." I wanted to

> *Leadership Lesson #1: Don't immediately take no for an answer even if you are moving away from what is considered the norm. Demonstrate the value of what you are trying to achieve.*

become a nurse because of the opportunities the profession offers, not simply to make money. I remember telling my parents that I wanted to get my bachelor's degree because I knew of the opportunities that would be available to me. After several discussions, my parents sat me down. "We will do what we can to support you financially for 4 years. At the end of your 4th year, it will be your sister's turn to go to college, and we can't support the two of you at the same time. If you don't finish in 4 years, you're on your own." I thought it was more than fair, and I will never be able to repay my parents for their decision.

Fast forward 10 years later, I eventually came to learn who Cherry Ames is (in case you don't know who she is, she's the nurse and central character of mystery novels published between 1942–1968 (Cherry Ames books in order [n.d.]). Cherry Ames—Student Nurse, Cherry Ames—Army Nurse, Cherry Ames—Cruise Nurse, and many more). While I did not have Cherry Ames to look up to as a child, nor many blood relatives who are nurses, there was no avoiding it. While going into nursing was a pragmatic decision, nursing runs through my veins, as I have grown up surrounded by the experiences and dedication of many Filipinx American nurses who came before me.

Nursing School, Here I Come!

The moment I walked onto the grounds of Mount St. Mary's University in Los Angeles, CA, I knew I had found the right place to call my home for the next 4 years. I submitted my college application for early admission and called the admissions counselor at least once a week to ask about my acceptance status. Finally, after excusing myself from art class, I was relieved to hear the news that I was accepted into Mount St. Mary's for the fall of 1995. I called my parents at work as soon as I got home and shared the great news. I could not contain my excitement and shared the news with family and friends. A family friend, a nurse for many years, said to me, "Why are you going into nursing? It's not a good field anymore. There are so many diseases like HIV. You're on your feet 12 hours a day." Another said, "Why are you going to that school? You don't need to go to a private school. You can just go to the community college for 2 years." Most were perplexed and said, "You don't need your bachelor's. We're all going to make the same money." I did not receive the support I thought I would get from the nurses who had been part of my life. There was no "Congratulations" or "Way to go!" or "I'm so glad you're going into nursing." I did not let this deter me and continued with my plan.

Mount St. Mary's was only an hour away, and I was relieved that my parents allowed me to move into on-campus housing. It did not take long for me to discover how ill-prepared I was for college, both academically and socially. I had to attend English tutoring sessions my freshman year. I was an introvert who was thrown into an environment that required me to put myself out there. I was lucky to have the support of a small, liberal arts women's college where I received the attention I needed to be successful.

Leadership Lesson #2: Bullying happens. Bullying knows no bounds—race, culture, socioeconomic status. Let the cycle end with you.

Soon enough, I started my clinical rotations. Reality shock and "eating your young" were phrases and conversations discussed with students early on, and the clinical rotations exposed me to the real world of nursing. Los Angeles had a large population of Filipinx nurses, and naturally, they were in every clinical rotation location I was assigned to. I met many of the *Titas* or aunties (what we call another woman who we know is a little older than we are as a sign of respect) along the way. My parents' advice echoed in my head as I began my clinical rotations—always be respectful, do what they say, don't create waves, be humble, put your head down, and work hard. So, if I did all these, I should not be a victim of the "eating your young" mentality. I was wrong. I arrived at the clinical site early on my first clinical day of junior year to give myself ample time to review my patient's chart. I was reading the patient information, but nervous about being in a new unit. "*Ano ba 'yan. Nandiyan na naman ang mga estudyante na ito. Pagulo lang. Kinukuha ang mga charts.*" Translation: "What is this? Here are these students again. They're just trouble. They're taking the charts." I happened to have the chart she was looking for.

> **Leadership Lesson #3: Demonstrate compassion for others so they may become their best self. Let others know you believe in them because your words might be just what they need to hear.**

I hesitated, not knowing how to respond. I turned around, handed her the chart, and said "*Tita, eto po 'yung chart ninyo. Sorry po.*" Translation: "Auntie, here's your chart. I'm sorry." She responded with "Ay, thank you." You see, the "eating your young" mentality transcends cultures. I would have thought that someone I have similarities with, someone with whom I "belong," would take care of me.

When I had an opportunity to attend hospital committee meetings, I wondered where the *Titas* were. In my 10 clinical rotations, not one *Tita* or *Tito* (uncle) held a leadership position. Were Filipinx nurses, who had the reputation for being caring, hardworking, and some of the best clinicians, only allowed to work at the point of care? Was this my destiny? Then, there was Mrs. Meyer. She was my leadership professor. She was a tall, slender woman with short, wavy, auburn hair. She was soft-spoken but spoke with authority. It was my last student–teacher conference ever, and I was excited and nervous because it was when I would receive my performance feedback as a student. She and I met at the cafeteria where we sat directly across from each other in a two-person booth. We chit-chatted a bit about how exciting it was for graduation to finally be here. She asked me about my plans after school. She said, "It's really important that when you meet people, you give a firm handshake," as she extended her right hand out to me over the table. I shook her hand and she said, "Let's try that again." After the third time, I was firm, and my handshake was approved. She then said something that has stuck with me and changed my perspective. She said, looking directly at me, "Larissa, you are smart and very capable. However, you are so timid and quiet I'm afraid people will not notice you and you will get lost in the shuffle." Mrs. Meyer, my last undergraduate nursing professor, changed my life. Her words were more than enough to boost my confidence. I knew then and there that I, too, could be a nurse leader. She was the one who made me realize that if I show up, do right, give thanks, I can make a difference..

Launch of A Nursing Career

The job market for nurses during my sophomore and junior years was bleak. "You better get your foot in the door, or you won't find a job," one recent new graduate said. What a scary thought! I was paying for a private education, and there was a chance I would not find a job after graduation. I applied for patient care services aide positions and was lucky enough to be hired at Children's Hospital Los Angeles.

During the last semester of my senior year, the hospital announced that all new graduate nurses were required to complete a 6-month RN Internship Program (transition to practice program). Wait a minute . . . I had just graduated from a baccalaureate program, I had been working in this organization for almost a year, and now I was required to go through a 6-month program? My unit manager said I had no choice. As a novice nurse, I knew what I knew and did not yet understand the value of a transition to practice program. After completing the RN Internship, I knew that I could not have made a better choice to launch my nursing career. I had a dedicated preceptor who showed me how to care for patients competently. I had a mentor who served as a sounding board when I struggled with skills like communicating with physicians. I met subject matter experts who taught me more than I ever expected. I had a group of new graduate nurses who, like me, were just dipping their toes in this world of pediatric nursing. And I soaked it all in.

Leadership Lesson #4: Your education never ends. There is always something new to learn even when you think you already know it.

The RN Internship started in July and culminated in December. What an exciting time that was! I was finally deemed to be ready for independent practice. Unfortunately, we were shorthanded during my first night shift. There were three new graduates, one RN who only worked at the hospital once a month, and the charge nurse. I was assigned a patient who had tetralogy of Fallot and had just completed his first of three surgeries. He was not doing well. The charge nurse checked on me several times during the night to see if I needed anything. As I was doing my midnight assessment, my little patient did not look so good. Something had changed in his breathing, his color, and his heart rate. I called the charge nurse immediately, and together we called the attending physician who, after assessing the patient, ordered for a transfer to the cardiothoracic ICU (CTICU) immediately. The charge nurse and I went with the CTICU team during the transfer. On our way back up to our unit, the charge nurse said, "You did good tonight. If it wasn't for your assessment skills, we would not have been able to transfer him so quickly." It was a tough night, but my charge nurse's comment boosted my self-confidence. Little by little, I was given more challenging assignments and more opportunities to improve my clinical skills.

Leadership Lesson #5: Meaningful recognition, no matter how small, gives confidence, hope, and makes one feel like they are part of a much larger vision than themselves.

As much as I enjoyed caring for the sickest patients, I started to notice that I was tired even at the beginning of the shift. I did not have time to recover from continuously caring for such high acuity patients shift after shift. I spoke with the charge nurse and requested to be assigned lesser acuity patients for a week to catch my breath. He did not say anything. The next day, all my patients had lower acuity and I was grateful. The next shift was the same. And the next. And the next. My new patient assignments made me feel like I had lost my team's trust, but I knew that I needed to have a mental and emotional break if I was to continue to care for my patients and their families competently.

An Opportunity That Opened Many Doors

A year and a half into my practice, I felt something was amiss. I had a desire for more, but I did not know what. It was too early in my career to think about any formal leadership role. I contemplated enrolling in graduate school to become a pediatric nurse practitioner. Then, a different opportunity came knocking on my door.

Leadership Lesson #6: Advocate for yourself. Each of us has a duty to ourselves to care for our emotional and mental well-being if we are to care for others.

"Curriculum Coordinator Position Available: RN Internship Program." I recall staring at the job opening posted on the whiteboard at the charge nurse's station for a few minutes. "Minimum education requirement: BSN," check. "Passionate about developing nurses," check. "Minimum years of nursing experience," wait— nothing was mentioned. I immediately sent an email to the curriculum coordinator for the program to inquire about the position. I learned about the plan to replicate the internship program at three additional pediatric facilities in Southern California and that two additional nurses were needed for the curriculum coordinator position. She encouraged

Leadership Lesson #7: Ignore the naysayers. The value of listening to feedback is critical. Learn how to distinguish the difference between feedback and cynicism.

me to apply even though I had only been a registered nurse for a year and a half, and I let my managers know of my intention to apply for the position. After the end of a shift a few days later, one of my managers and I happened to walk out together. We started making conversation, and then she said, "If I were the person interviewing you, I wouldn't hire you. You're too new. You don't have a lot of experience yet." I was stunned. All I remember saying was, "Thank you for the feedback. I will let you know how it goes."

> *Leadership Lesson #8: Don't be afraid to try something new even if it seems out of reach. The worst thing that can happen is they say no. You are a nurse. You have endless opportunities.*

I remember a few of the interview questions: "Having gone through the internship yourself, what would you change?" "What was the best part about being in the internship?" "How do you feel about videoconferencing?" I did not know what videoconferencing was and after asking the interviewers to explain it, I was excited about a new technology that would allow us to broadcast the classes to other organizations. After three rounds of interviews with different groups, I received the good news. I was offered the part-time, grant-funded coordinator position, which became a full-time role a month later.

I was excited to start in my position. My first assignment, however, was not so exciting, but was an important part of the whole transition to practice experience. The graduation for the next cohort of new graduates was near, and I was handed a slide carousel with about 80 slides of different events throughout the program. My assignment was to time the progression of the slide image with appropriate music. 1 ... 2 ... 3 ... 4 ... 5 ... click ... 1 ... 2 ... 3 ... 4 ... 5 ... click. My immediate thought was that there had to be a better way to use my skills to support the educational experience for learners. For the first couple of months, I observed, learned the current processes and structures, and asked questions. I proposed opportunities for enhancement once I felt comfortable in my role and responsibilities. One challenge we had was that subject matter experts (SMEs) did not always show up to teach the class they had agreed to. I discovered that sending email reminders and an agenda was not enough. My emails were getting buried in the hundreds of emails they already had in their inbox. I decided that I needed to be in front of them. I carried copies of the daily class agendas around with me wherever I went. My weekly routine was to deliver the daily class agenda for the following week to each SME. Each class agenda had the name, date, time, and class highlighted for each SME. If they were not in their offices and the door was locked, I slipped the paper under their door. If I ran into them in the hallway or cafeteria, I handed them the agenda personally. "You are tenacious, I will give you that," said one SME. I developed relationships with each one. I got to know them, and they got to know me. When I needed help, someone was always there to help. I became friends with the environmental services team, and when I needed doors to be unlocked or tables to be brought into the meeting, it was a nonissue. I enjoyed working with each subject matter expert as we transferred their transparencies or slides into PowerPoint (which was new at that

> *Leadership Lesson #9:*
> *Build relationships.*
> *No one person can do*
> *anything alone.*

time). Together, we learned how to best use a new innovative technology. We were all in this journey together.

I learned many new concepts, ideas, strategies, processes, and skills in my new role. I had learned the importance of mentoring during the RN Internship, where I was assigned a mentor who walked me through scenarios and role-played situations I was either unfamiliar with or needed some coaching on. I was fortunate to have many nursing leaders who mentored me along the way. I never felt alone. I found my second mentor when I went through the same situation with implementing the videoconferencing capability for the RN Internship. I was in an unfamiliar space. I needed direction and guidance on how to use the system but, more importantly, on getting buy-in from the team. She opened her door when I needed someone to share ideas with and allowed me to express frustrations when I felt stuck.

> *Leadership Lesson #10:*
> *Find mentors who can*
> *assist in your development.*
> *Find a person with whom*
> *you can share the good*
> *and the ugly without*
> *judgment.*

A second opportunity came almost a year into my role of curriculum coordinator. The program manager position became available, and I was encouraged to apply. I was nervous and eager to take on this new role. Aside from leading committee meetings during college, this was my first exposure to having a formal leadership role. I observed various team members around the table during meetings. I watched each person's demeanor. I saw what was effective and what was not. I intentionally listened more than I spoke. I wanted to develop my communication skills, but first, I needed to learn the practice of active listening. I took notes in every meeting—lots of them. My notes reflected the conversations, questions I had, and potential solutions to the problem statement. I learned how to integrate ideas. I drew workflows during meetings to help me understand what was happening. I learned strategies such as asking the five whys to clarify the problem statement (Whiteman et al., 2021). I also learned that it's okay to not have all the answers.

These skills were not only new for me but beyond my cultural comfort zone. There are certain sets of expectations for a Filipina woman, such as refraining from challenging the status quo, abstaining from being too assertive, and leaving the decisions to the higher-ups. I was taught that whatever the boss says, goes.

Leadership Lesson #11: Develop your listening and communication skills. Listen for understanding instead of listening to prepare your response. Clarify, verify, and amplify. Be comfortable when you do not have all the answers and admit that you do not, but follow through with finding out the answers or directing the person to where they can find the answer.

I knew I was starting to break traditions and expectations. I was beginning to find my stride in my role as a program manager when the meeting that would propel my career beyond my greatest ambition would happen.

"I Need You to Attend This Meeting"

"Larissa, come to a meeting in the 3 East Conference Room at
10:00 a.m. No need to prepare for anything. Just come and bring
the preceptor, mentor, debriefer, and SME manuals." I walked into
the meeting room, not knowing what to expect, and found my
team having a lively conversation with a gentleman I had never
met before. The meeting started with brief introductions and then,
oh my . . . the 2-hour meeting was way over my head. It seemed as
if everyone was speaking a different language. By the end, everyone was excited about the possibility of . . . I had no idea what. I
spoke with my direct supervisor separately to clarify the purpose of
the meeting and my role. As a summary, the meeting was just the
beginning of what would eventually evolve into what is now Versant Healthcare Competency Solutions®.

I spent the next 6 months learning about new education platforms, new technologies and creating workflows to describe the
activities involved in implementing an RN Internship. I met with
at least half a dozen learning management system (LMS) vendors
to investigate whether there was already a solution in the market
that met our needs. In every meeting, I found myself wondering
whether it made sense to build our own system instead. I gave my
feedback to the leaders making the decision on which LMS to purchase. Eventually, the team decided that it would be best to build
our own system, and I was elated! Imagine—we would build something from the ground up and this had never been done before. We
had the ability to create a system to mirror the activities of preceptors, unit managers, new graduates, SMEs, mentors, and debriefers.
I worked directly with the systems engineers to design the original version of Voyager, the web-based platform currently in use
to manage the intricacies of implementing a systems approach to

workforce development. I served as a conduit between the systems engineers and the team at the hospital. I relayed the feedback the key stakeholders had about Voyager and vice versa.

Our timeline of 12 months was sped up when we signed our first client (mind you, we did not yet have a product to show), and we had to have everything ready 3 months earlier than originally planned. I was fortunate to have an experienced nurse executive working alongside me who provided the guidance and the direction for creating new processes and structures to ensure that the program is replicable and scalable while maintaining standards for success. We updated the current and created new reference materials through the holidays, and when Voyager finally went live, everyone (including me) was nervous. We collected metrics from the new graduates in the program, and they entered their answers in Voyager. The new graduates completed the paper version of the metrics first and then transcribed their answers into the system—we did not trust the technology. Like many new

> *Leadership Lesson #12: Never give up. Sometimes the situation is a temporary setback. If you understand the problem you are trying to solve, there is always an opportunity to create an innovative solution.*

systems, there were kinks along the way. I remember one training I conducted for the unit managers and most of the navigation bars were not working. At that moment, it felt like every navigation bar I clicked on resulted in an error message. My co-trainer contacted the system engineer while I continued to discuss how to use the system using the reference materials with screenshots. How do you trust technology that does not consistently work during training? I was nervous most of the time because I never knew what would happen. We made changes to the engineering team, which resolved the technology issues. The system began running smoothly and subsequently garnered a Microsoft award. The key stakeholders became more comfortable with the system as they continued to use it.

One of the most difficult parts for me during this time was that I knew I was spending almost all my efforts with the new client, and there was still a cohort of new graduate nurses back home who needed me. My team was gracious enough to cover for me, but I was still the program manager. When I conducted a focus group midway through the cohort, I heard it all: me not being there for them, the system being clunky, and the internship not running smoothly. There was nothing I could do but listen and acknowledge what was happening. I apologized and promised that the situation would improve. I met with my supervisor and recommended that we hire a new program manager. We could not possibly replicate the program successfully elsewhere if we were failing at home.

Calculated Risks

I hired my replacement as the program manager at the hospital without a guarantee of a job because the new company was not fully approved. "It's okay," I told myself. "I'm a nurse and if things don't work out, there is always something for me." Of course, this wasn't a decision I made on my own since I was newly married. My husband and I discussed the pros and cons of taking a role in a start-up company. He said, "I will support you in whatever decision you make, but if you don't at least try, you will regret it. You're a nurse and if things don't work out, there are other opportunities for you." That's not all, now I had to explain all this to my parents. A start-up company with no guarantees, a new role which required travel to other states and staying in hotels on my own, going to places I had never been. A nurse works in a hospital. A nurse means security. Why would I want to leave a job that was secure and in one of the premier pediatric institutions in the nation? As worried as they were, my parents supported my decision. Almost 2 decades later, these questions still comes up: "What do you mean you don't work at a hospital?" "You don't work weekends and holidays?" "You don't have more than one job?" "You're a travel nurse?" A career path of joining a start-up company and becoming an entrepreneur is not common among Filipinx nurses and still requires explanation from time to time.

In less than a year from when the idea was conceived about the need to develop a way to scale the program implementation, my hard work had come to fruition. Between the announcement of a new company and my formal transition into the role, I was introduced to the art of negotiation.

As a woman, especially a minority woman, gender bias is an obstacle we must learn to navigate because we, along with our other colleagues, face increasing responsibilities and expectations. As nurses, we learned that we need to advocate for our

Leadership Lesson #13: Learn the art of negotiation.

patients and for ourselves, but I do not remember any class about negotiations, especially when it comes to salaries. I did not have a formal education around the art of negotiation, so I met with a few unit leaders to ask them for advice. My emotions were all over the place because some of the unit leaders were concerned not about the salary but whether this new venture would be a good move for my career. Some did provide me with recommendations on how to approach negotiating my salary. I had to be clear on my target salary, what salary I would be willing to accept, and when I would walk away from the negotiation. Two decades later, I would learn that the process I used is knowing your Best Alternative to a Negotiated Agreement, or BATNA (Negotiation Experts, n.d.).

A Whole New Territory

I spent the next 5 years implementing the RN Internship, now known as the RN Residency, at hospitals nationwide. This gave me a new perspective on health care around the country—especially similarities and differences in approaches around workforce development. Opportunities to present in small and large groups became more available, and I came to realize consulting as an entrepreneur is not much different from being a healthcare leader. One must know their audience, group dynamics, and have a clear understanding of the organization's strategic goals, just to name a few. What was new to me were things such as business dinner etiquette and where to sit in a meeting room. One needs to know where the power seat is and that the opposite end is the second power position. The flanking positions are those next to the top two power seats, and they have the ear of the power positions. Who knew that where you sit in a meeting room matters!

As I met nurse leaders across the country during my business travels, I often was asked about my plans to go back to school. I always responded with, "I don't know yet. I don't know if this is the right time. I just had a baby." The answer I heard over and over was, "There will never be the right time." When an even bigger change in my career happened 5 years later, once Versant

Advantage, LLC, separated from Children's Hospital Los Angeles and became what is now Versant Holdings, LLC, I could no longer contemplate whether I should go back to school. It was a necessary step if I was to have an impactful role in this healthcare space. I decided to get my master's in business administration because in today's environment, understanding the business of health care is a requirement. As a new mother in a position where I was traveling for work often, I knew I could not do it alone. I depended on my husband to care for our son while I traveled and completed all my schoolwork ahead of time as much as I could. I was forced to elevate my time management and prioritization skills. I blocked off Sunday afternoons for reading, completing assignments, and writing papers at a coffee shop nearby so that I could spend the rest of the weeknights with my family. I also leveraged having a team who had the expertise in areas I was studying, such as finance and statistics. The nurse leaders who had encouraged me to go back to school were right—there will never be the right time. As challenging as it was juggling multiple responsibilities, I enjoyed being in school because I was able to directly apply what I was learning to what I was doing. The challenge for most students is that they receive the knowledge but may not always understand the practice. Since my work responsibilities and school were aligned, it

> *Leadership Lesson #14: Be willing to explore your potential by taking personal risk. Give yourself permission to make mistakes. Learn from it and move on. Do not let the mistake define who you are as a leader.*

was easier to translate knowledge to practice. If I were to summarize how my MBA continues to benefit me it would be that (1) I learned strategic consulting skills valuable for our organization and for our client partners, (2) my MBA expanded my perspective around how to approach the challenges we have in this business of health care, and (3) my MBA helped me hone my skills and abilities to integrate ideas and form strategic solutions.

Like many company acquisitions, some people were brought along into the new company, and some were not. My title stayed the same, but not for long. One by one, the top leadership of the company found other opportunities. I was thrust into the role of leading a team full of seasoned, passionate, and strong-willed nurses as the assistant vice president. I knew how to implement the program like the back of my hand. What I did not know was how to lead, manage, and grow a team. I sought out mentors both internally and externally, and like many, I made mistakes along the way. A year into our venture, additional changes brought me into the top leadership position as the vice president and chief operating officer, and eventually as president a short time later. "It's lonely at the top, you know," I remember one of the other team executives saying to me while driving from a client site to the airport. I sat in the passenger seat of the car quietly trying to absorb the moment. I thought about what I heard for days and decided that it would only be "lonely at the top" if I allowed it. I thought about what I could do to engage my team members in decision-making and collaborating on strategies. I may be the person providing the direction and the vision for the organization, but my team operationalizes that vision. My vision for creating an integrated workforce retention and practice solution was realized when Versant's competency-based system was released. I am fortunate that my managing partner gives me the autonomy and the authority to elevate our transition to practice program as part of a solution that addresses the fragmentation in health care.

As I continued to be exposed and introduced to nurse leaders I had admired from afar, professional and healthcare community engagement became a goal I focused on. I sought out new learning opportunities such as completing Cornell University's Women in Leadership Certificate Program. I created short- and long-term goals for myself. One of those goals was to volunteer for a local or national healthcare board. Serving on a board is an important role, and I prepared myself for the commitment. I read resources on what it means to be a board member, the role and responsibilities, and strategies for success such as engaging with others during and after meetings, coming prepared, and actively participating. I learned about the competencies necessary for a board member—leadership experience, industry experience, financial expertise, corporate governance, and strategy development. I examined my areas of strength and weakness. I found mentors and read additional resources to develop skills that were not quite at the level where I wanted them to be. I wrote down specific goals I had for development and shared them with select individuals from my network. I hired an executive coach to further assist me with developing my personal and professional objectives, provide another perspective, and act as my sounding board.

When I was approached by a nonprofit organization to become part of their board, I did not immediately agree to do so because I wanted to make sure I was a right fit and that my skills were what they needed. I spent an hour with the president of the organization learning about their goals, strategies, and what she thought I could contribute. It did not take me long to agree to the commitment. My approach with another organization in which I am currently a member of the board of directors was different. I learned that a board member recently stepped down, which meant that there was a board position open. I reached out to my contact and asked about the needs of the board. I knew that my skills would be a match. I submitted my curriculum vitae for consideration, and I was voted in a couple of months later. Attending my first board meeting was nerve-wracking, especially after everyone introduced themselves during the meeting. The board consisted of well-published and well-known leaders in health care. Sometimes, there are moments I question myself and ask whether I belong. When this happens, I reach out to the board leaders to ask for feedback on my performance, which always makes me feel at ease.

> *Leadership Lesson #15: Make a point to seek feedback and ask for specific information. Write your opportunities for improvement, and be specific in your goals. If you write them, they will be harder to ignore.*

Another goal I established for myself is sharing my expertise with the community. I spoke at a local middle school about the nursing profession and mentored new graduates (nursing and non-nursing) in résumé-building and interviewing skills. Sharing what the nursing profession is and all the possibilities that come with it is one of the most enjoyable moments in my career. I showed videos of flight nurses and detailed how nurses contributed during disasters. I had the middle schoolers pick from a set of pictures who they thought the nurses were—a woman in a suit, a woman in scrubs, a man in scrubs holding an infant, a man in front of a computer, a woman in a lab coat with a stethoscope around her neck. The "ooohs" and "aahhhs" after I revealed that all the people on the screen are nurses made me feel like I met my objective for the day—to impress upon them that nurses come in many different forms and they can be one too. I showed them how to feel their pulse, then made them do jumping jacks and count their pulse right after. Although preparing for the presentation always took time, and it was always a whole day event, the smile and excitement I saw on their faces was immeasurable. The same smile and excitement I saw on new graduates' faces when

Leadership Lesson #16: Giving back gives us a higher purpose. Give back in any form you can. No one is in a better and more unique position than we are as nurses to contribute back to our profession and make a difference in health care.

they were hired into their first jobs, and it gave me the same feeling of contentment. I once attended a wedding where I sat next to a couple and the woman was a new graduate nurse. She was nervous about applying for jobs. After talking all night, I told her to email me her résumé and I could give her feedback. Soon after we finished working on her résumé, she called and asked about how to prepare for an interview. We talked through what questions she might possibly be asked, and I recommended strategies on how to answer them. I remember receiving a very excited call when I was at a client site. She told me she had been offered a position and that she would not have been able to do it without my help.

A Brighter Future . . . Growing New Leaders

As nurse leaders, we learn different strategies on how to be an effective leader. The vast number of resources and information available can be daunting. However important it is to learn about leadership styles, I knew I would have to find my own leadership style aligned with my true north. I integrated all that I had learned in the last 2 decades into three competencies that define my leadership style: competence, compassion, and courage. Competence to do my job well, compassion for those around me to help others be their best selves, and courage, especially in times of adversity, to do what is right. These three competencies have served me well—as a woman, as a mother, as Filipinx, and as an entrepreneur and leader.

In every situation, I make a habit of celebrating little wins for 15 minutes and then spending hours to evaluate where the opportunities are. With my work at Versant Healthcare Competency Solutions, I have been fortunate to have data to direct where opportunities are in improving the nursing workforce. Data and outcomes are the great equalizer—we know we can't manage what we can't measure. Nurses are in an invaluable position to improve the profession, health, and health care. There is an opportunity to demonstrate how data and outcomes contribute to the betterment of our profession.

My induction as a fellow into the American Academy of Nursing gives me an additional platform to contribute to the growth of future nurse leaders and facilitate the role minority nurses play in improving health care in the United States. We have an opportunity to highlight contributions of Asian American nurses in leadership roles to forge the path for others earlier in their careers. We must educate the Asian American community about contributions of Asian American nurses. We must serve as mentors and introduce minority nurses to career pathways that they may not know exist and the endless possibilities within the nursing profession.

My journey as a nurse leader and as an entrepreneur may be unusual. I know that I have had to overcome many gender and cultural barriers along the way. A mentor once told me that if you walk in the room like you own it, then you own it. I learned that if you want a seat at the table, then do not sit in a chair by the wall. If there are no empty chairs around the table, find one and ask for space to bring your chair in.

> *Leadership Lesson #17: As leaders, we must be leaders early in our careers, then be a leader every step of the way.*

Often, we are told that as nurses, we must find our voice. On the contrary, I believe that each of us already has that voice inside. We all have stories to tell about who we are as individuals and as nurses. What we need to do is embrace it. Once we have done that, we must own it. Then, we must lead with it every step of the way.

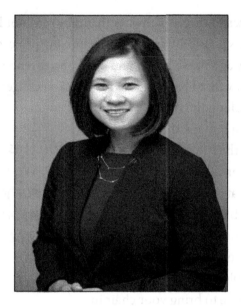

Larissa Africa, MBA, BSN, RN, FAAN

Larissa Africa is the president of Versant Healthcare Competency Solutions™ and is responsible for its strategic and operational leadership. Larissa has spent 2 decades implementing, managing, and leading strategies to develop nursing organizations. Larissa has developed a competency-based nurse residency program, one that is considered a gold standard in the industry. As a pioneer in the transition to practice space, she led the deployment of a competency-based model that integrates and standardizes nursing workforce development across the entire healthcare continuum, addressing high-demand areas such as long-term care, home health, and advanced practice nursing. Larissa's collective body of work continues to change the landscape of how healthcare organizations integrate and sustain workforce retention and practice solutions. Larissa holds a bachelor of science in nursing from Mount

St. Mary's University, a master's degree in business administration: health care management from University of Phoenix, and an Executive Women in Leadership certificate through Cornell University. She is an author of numerous highly recognized publications and book chapters, a national and international speaker, and a member of the American Organization for Nursing Leadership's Foundation board of directors. Larissa was inducted as a fellow into the American Academy of Nursing in 2021.

3

Unbeatable Determination

Frank Baez, BS, RN

My name is Frank Baez, and I am an experienced health-care professional—a former hospital housekeeper, an NYU graduate, and now a bilingual ICU nurse.

I was born in the Dominican Republic and immigrated to the United States as a teen in 2004 with my two siblings to reunite with my mom and late grandfather in Brooklyn, New York. Over the next several years, I worked in a hospital and was able to advance into new roles and work assignments, gaining increasing responsibility along the way. While employed, I mastered the English language, graduated from Sheepshead Bay High School, and earned an associate's degree and two bachelor's degrees.

In 2006, at the age of 17, I started working as a weekend housekeeper at NYU Langone's Tisch Hospital. Four years later, I became a patient transporter and consequently a unit clerk. My interest in the medical field grew at NYU Langone. I applied for a unit clerk position in the Special Care Unit in the Orthopedic Hospital because I wanted to work directly with patients. Although the idea of nursing was constantly in my mind, it wasn't until a pivotal incident occurred that the thought was brought to fruition. While working as a unit clerk, there was a patient who had experienced a cardiopulmonary arrest, and I noticed not only how the nurse advocated for the patient, but also how diligently she worked with members of the interprofessional team to save this patient's life. She entrusted me to deliver critical lab work to the laboratory for this patient. Something as tiny as delivering a lab test while taking in all that information, observing the incident myself, was transformative—and in that moment, I knew that nursing was my calling. I wanted to embody the qualities and attributes similar to the nurse who advocated for the patient during the cardiopulmonary resuscitation.

While working in the hospital, I earned my associate degree from the Borough of Manhattan Community College and bachelors of arts in spanish literature and biological science from Hunter College. I graduated from Hunter with a 2.8 GPA, which I feel did not reflect my full potential, but was a direct result of double majoring and juggling work and school. Not only was I working during the week in the evenings as a patient transporter in the hospital, but on the weekends, I was also working as a waiter to support my education and my family.

> *In that moment, I knew that nursing was my calling.*

Through these challenging obstacles, the realization dawned on me that balancing school and financial demands can have a negative impact on your academic success, even if you are trying to support yourself and your loved ones. But I didn't let this stop my drive. After graduating from Hunter, I went back to school to take higher level Spanish and biology courses, as well as the nursing prerequisites to improve my GPA and to prove not only to a college but to myself that I was capable of academic success and able to handle the rigor of a nursing program.

After almost 12 years of working in a hospital setting, I decided to take the plunge into the medical field. I felt ready to expand my knowledge and go back to school to pursue an accelerated bachelor of science in nursing at NYU Rory Meyers College of Nursing (NYU Meyers). Once I completed the prerequisites, I applied to NYU Meyers. At the beginning, when I applied to the program, I was unsure about my acceptance due to the highly competitive nursing program and my abysmal GPA, but I overcame my fear and pushed forward. When the senior director of nursing at NYU Langone Orthopedic Hospital found out I had intentions of applying to nursing school, she offered to write me a letter of recommendation. I believe the exquisite letter of recommendation, my academic performance and improvement, and my work experience were the necessary ingredients, and I was accepted into the Accelerated Bachelor of Science in Nursing program at NYU.

I was beyond ecstatic when I received the news! The memory of that day is ingrained in my head. I was at work when I noticed an email from the NYU Office of Admissions. I excused myself to the break room because I didn't want anyone to see me crying if it wasn't the outcome I wanted. I prepared myself to cry, grabbing a napkin while opening my phone, but the email wouldn't load for what seemed like eternity. I became desperate and started swiping up and down in exasperation until finally the email loaded. I couldn't believe my eyes. I ran outside, nervous and in disbelief, and asked one of my colleagues to read the email for me. She confirmed that I was accepted! I was so excited that words couldn't describe all the emotions I was feeling that day. I then called my mother, my manager, and the director of nursing and told them immediately about my acceptance. They were all equally excited and happy for me. I took the letter from one floor to the next to tell all my friends that I was accepted into nursing school. News quickly spread through the hospital from the PACU to the OR and even the outpatient clinics at the Orthopedic Hospital. I never knew that I had so many friends who were all rooting for me!

After surviving the emotional rollercoaster, the reality of my acceptance into nursing school weighed heavily on me. The question of how I was going to pay for nursing school threatened to overshadow my excitement. NYU is a private world-class university with a high tuition cost, but because I was working in the hospital full-time, I was able to take advantage of the tuition reimbursement benefits offered by the employee union. The union would cover my full tuition for the first two semesters if I was working full time, but to be able to receive the reimbursement benefits, you have to be able to pay for the semester yourself out of pocket ahead of time; then, the union would reimburse you at the end of the semester once you successfully passed all of your courses. I applied for a student loan with my mom to be able to afford the first semester of school. In addition, another blessing came my way: NYU Langone Orthopedic Hospital awarded me the non-nurses scholarship during Nurses Week.

With each successive semester, the union reduced the amount of financial aid I received to a percentage basis instead of full tuition in order to accommodate other members. I also had to reduce my hours at the hospital because the workload of school and work had become overwhelming. The nurse manager of the Special Care Unit at that time was tremendously accommodating to my schedule and allowed me to float to other units as well as exchange shifts and schedules with other unit clerks from nearby units within the same facility. This allowed me the opportunity to attend school and not miss classes or clinicals while also and maintaining my professional role. Such incredible teamwork—and support from everyone at all levels of the organization—gave me the opportunity to study the career of my dreams while working to sustain myself and continuing to help my family at the same time.

One of the many programs I took advantage of during nursing school was the mentorship program. In this program, I was paired with a peer advisor who guided me through my classes and taught me how to navigate nursing school. NYU also provided me with books and resources to help me learn the material. My mentor met with me once a month, communicated via email and text messages, closely monitored my progress through my courses, and was available for anything that I needed, whether it was tutoring or a phone call to explain a subject. This experience was crucial in the process of getting through nursing school.

During my last semester of nursing school, I had to cut down my hours to part time to focus on my final obstacle: the board exam for licensure known as the NCLEX. Thankfully, the school provided additional courses to help students practice and be well equipped to pass the licensing test. Graduation day was a dream come true. So many of my coworkers attended the commencement ceremony held at Yankee Stadium in New York City. So many people had helped me to earn a bachelor of science degree with a major in nursing. My nursing career could now begin!

Upon graduation, I was awarded the Daisy Award for Extraordinary Nursing Students and qualified for the position of a staff nurse in the Cardiothoracic Intensive Care Unit at NYU Langone Health. My next goal is to obtain a doctor of nursing practice (DNP) degree that will help me to function at the highest levels of nursing practice. My ultimate goal is to help improve and advance the health care of minority groups who live in underserved communities in the city of New York and have little to no access to health care.

As an immigrant coming from a disadvantaged population and as a nurse who worked in the COVID-19 intensive care unit, I have been able to personally see and experience the challenges that vulnerable communities face. It has always been a goal of mine to climb the ladder and make a real difference in health care. Throughout my journey as a housekeeper, patient transporter, and unit clerk, I was able to see patients in their most vulnerable states of being. I witnessed how nurses interacted with their patients, many of whom were critically ill. These life-changing experiences were what ultimately inspired me to apply to the BS program at NYU Rory Meyers College of Nursing and what motivate me every day working as a nurse at NYU Langone—often walking the same hallways as I did many years ago to transport patients or deliver labs.

> *Throughout my journey as a housekeeper, patient transporter, and unit clerk, I was able to see patients in their most vulnerable states of being.*

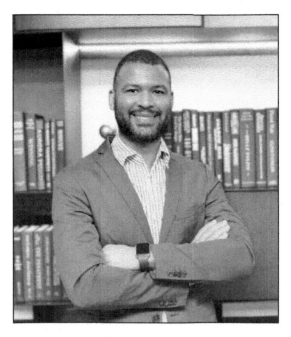

Frank Baez, BSN, RN

Frank Baez has worked in the healthcare industry for more than 14 years since he first started at NYU Langone Health as a house-keeper. He is currently a registered nurse in the Cardiothoracic Intensive Care Unit (CTICU) in the same hospital. Frank, inspired by his colleagues and supported by the leadership of NYU Langone Health, became interested in pursuing a meaningful career in nursing. He is particularly drawn to critical care and bridging the gaps in health disparities of vulnerable populations. Frank is a member of the New York City Men in Nursing, the American Nurses Association, and the National Association of Hispanic Nurses.

4

I Can, I Will, I Must

Judith Cullinane, PhD, MSN, RN, CAGS, CCRN-K

Why Did You Choose Nursing as a Career?

In 1985, I was working at a community clinic when one of the nurses approached me and said, "You should be a nurse. You love the health science and know it well. You also connect with people in a loving way." She was a pediatric nurse, and I adored how children connected to her and how adolescents would confide in and trust her with some of their challenges. Often, she would walk me through some of the diagnoses, treatments, and ways nurses helped patients heal. Our discussions led me to explore the opportunity to attend a college for nursing and to explore ways to reenter college, since I had recently graduated and finances to attend a second college were limited.

This nurse was a pillar of strength for many in the community. She understood the challenges of growing up in an urban setting, and most of all, she knew how to use the experience to provide drive and motivation. She capitalized on moments to point out the beauty, essence, and value of the Hispanic community and culture. Her honesty and kindness were seen by many as guidance.

Describe Your Admission to a Nursing Program

During the 1980s era, bridge and accelerated nursing programs were in discussion but not yet developed, and given my financial situation, I selected and attended an associate degree in nursing (ADN) program in Boston. My admission process went well; however, I did find myself to be an *N* of one—I was the only Latina in the program.

I do not remember much transcultural education in my nursing program at that time, nor do I remember anyone exploring different ways in which to manage the healing process of those with different beliefs, values, or preferences. Often, as the *N* of one, I was asked to translate in my clinical practicum as a student. All who asked were often very grateful of my help. However, I would also hear nurses discuss at times the need of a translator as a nuisance, and without much thought, they would make comments that were biased or that insinuated stereotyping. Initially, I perceived or simply wrote off these comments as just someone being angry in life. It took me about 10 years in the profession to step forward and redirect or correct the negative views with confidence.

> *I did find myself to be an N of one— I was the only Latina in the program.*

Progression and Challenges in the Program

I progressed through the program well academically. My challenges related more to perceptions of not being intellectual enough, stereotyping and believing I had an appearance too ornate for nursing, or even just being marginalized because I was an *N* of one and different. It is here where I found myself being judged. My perception was that there was lack of confidence in my ability, regardless of my grades. I often would encounter more questioning in the classroom or in the clinical setting and even nonverbal behavior that suggested they were thinking, "How could she possibly be that smart?" Unlike most individuals, these actions tended to silently motivate me rather than cause me to distance myself. They fueled me internally to be the best I could be in caring for people. I processed and entrenched myself in the experiences and the learning component of caring for the ill and their families. Through these actions, I became the nurse scientist I am today.

Share About Your First Job and Your Career Progression

My first couple of jobs as a clinical nurse were very interesting, and probably in hindsight, they were the nursing roles that drove me to do what I do today. I started on a cardiac stepdown unit and then transferred after 8 months to a pediatric intensive care unit (PICU). This was one of the first new-graduate nurse orientation pilots done at the organization in this setting, and I remember how honored I was to have been chosen. My only nay say is how I was told that being bilingual really helped me clinch the opportunity. At the time, I do remember asking myself whether this was the only reason I was hired. I again felt a sense of not belonging. Although the statement was probably not meant to be insulting, it did make me wonder. The comment of "being Hispanic clinched it for you" silently resonated and troubled me for a very long time.

The cardiac stepdown unit experience provided me with exceptional fundamental knowledge of the cardiac system and in turn, the experience provided me with the necessary skills for systems thinking, critical thinking, and sound clinical judgment necessary in nursing. In the PICU, I had the privilege of having one of the most experienced nurses in the field of pediatrics, as well as being one of the most organized and disciplined individuals. She served as my preceptor during the orientation period and for confidentiality, I will refer to her as Louise in the storyline.

Louise had been a nurse for about 20 years when we met, and she had a military background. She was incredibly knowledgeable and poised. Her characteristics, organized way of being, and true can-do attitude were traits that I could identify with very well. Not once did she ever make me feel inept or unqualified. Our days together began with confidence, and I always felt that my questions were answered and recommendations appreciated. These are days that I often reflect upon. The key word is "confidence." Her ability to continuously make me feel heard and empowered gave me the ability to continue and build strength and resiliency to embrace unknowns and lifelong learning. Later in my career, I embedded the statement "I can, I will, I must" into my thoughts and practice. Most often now, I find myself using it to motivate others.

Challenges

Many of my challenges throughout my career as a Latina nurse have been related to feeling marginalized or stereotyped. Assumptions or untruths of people of color or of different backgrounds are often the platforms that cause racism, marginalization, and biases. Although Louise did a wonderful job precepting me, I often found difficulty in finding my voice to speak up for myself and others when it came to these untruths. It was hard at times, and I lived two separate lives during that time: the life of a nurse with other nurses and clinicians and the life of me at home, with family and friends.

Fast-forward to having 10 years of experience and having moved over into the world of neonatal intensive clinical care, and I can remember the self-change I experienced that made me find my voice. I remember a conversation where assumptions were being made about a teenage mother. The judgment and criticism being made of the individual stirred me up inside, and I recall turning around and asking the nurses present how they came to the conclusions they were discussing. I used analogies and examples of how off base they were in their interpretation of the teenage mother's behavior and found myself explaining how important it was to recognize and stop their hurtful assumptions. While many remained silent as I spoke, others asked questions, and I began to see subtle changes in their behavior toward this mother. More so, I saw a difference when new teenage mothers came in to see their babies. I saw

Assumptions or untruths of people of color or of different backgrounds are often the platforms that cause racism, marginalization, and biases.

there can be progress toward a better understanding of different cultures and people of color. Hope is important to maintain.

Opportunities

The biggest opportunity for me as I progressed through my nursing career has been finding a voice to educate others. My biggest concern remains the lack of knowledge across the profession about the difficulties for people of color, both in the profession and as students. There is a tendency to point the finger at an organization to make a change, but my belief is that an organization is made of people and that it is the people who make the change. If each could simply pause to reflect on the inaccuracies of their views, then a catalyst of change would occur. Being impacted by financial constraints or limited in English proficiency does not imply lack of intelligence or capability. There needs to be better academic counseling and guidance for building confidence in students around choosing and succeeding in the profession of nursing from entry into school to advancement in a career.

Current Role

Through determination, I have progressed to the role of associate chief nursing officer for nursing research, innovation, professional development, and nursing quality. I completed a PhD degree in Healthcare Professions. I believe I am well prepared for the role. My commitment to diversify my knowledge, skills, and abilities has ensured that I am competent in the role and have

"I can, I will, I must."

proficient skills in leadership and expertise to carry out the necessary responsibilities.

Challenges

The challenge in reaching this level of nursing was having to prove my abilities a little more than usual. However, now I make note to attribute the experiences to a learning journey mapping the essence of my resiliency, how to see beyond and how to believe, and that yes, "I can, I will, I must."

Opportunities

A big opportunity for me in this role is to publish and present not only my story but also my contributions and suggestions for the future of nursing.

Your Recommendations for Equity in the Future

Recent societal events have exposed many inequities. The first step to progress is discussion and leaning in to discover, to understand, to accept, and to respect each other. My recommendation for equity in the future is to continue with purposeful steps and measures for building knowledge and skills in diversity, equity, and inclusion. This topic is multifaceted with many intersectional concepts. As a profession, we should capitalize on the great works by others to help people understand how to embrace differences in others, use reflection techniques to ensure a personal check on biases, create forums and hold discussions on all viewpoints, and then facilitate a collegial consensus. It is a beginning, and the beginning steps create foundational platforms that acknowledge all we have learned (truths, untruths, or vagueness) while moving toward a better place, no matter the difficulty.

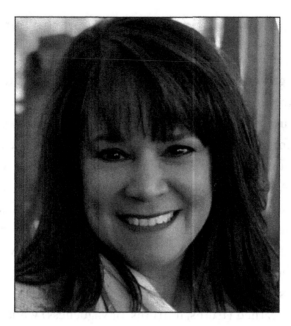

Judith Cullinane, PhD, MSN, RN, CAGS, CCRN-K

Judi is a graduate from the schools of nursing at Caritas Laboure, Boston, MA; Graceland University in Independence, MO; and Simmons University, Boston, MA, where she obtained her PhD. She is the associate chief nursing officer of the Robin and David Jaye Center for Nursing Excellence at Tufts Medical Center and Tufts Children's Hospital. She is also an adjunct associate professor of nursing practice at Simmons University and an adjunct associate professor at Tufts University, School of Medicine and School of Public Health. She has been acknowledged by the International Nurses Association as a nurse leader and serves as a commissioner of the American Association Credentialing Center for Nursing Continuous Professional Development. She has served on several boards, including the National Nursing Advisory Board for Becton

Dickinson; the Organization of Nurse Leaders in MA, CT, NH, RI, VT; the Massachusetts Action Coalition Campaign for the Future of Nursing; the Nurse of the Future Core Competencies Committee; and the Culture of Health and the Diversity Advisory Council. She is the past president for Sigma Theta Tau, Theta at Large Chapter 007 and the past president of the Massachusetts "Boston" Chapter of the National Association of Hispanic Nurses.

5

A Space for Everyone: Visibility in Nursing Through Service, Mentorship, and Leadership

Sasha DuBois, MSN, RN

Why Did You Choose Nursing as a Career?

I come from a family of service: nurses, teachers, judges, police officers. My maternal great-great-grandfather was an immigrant from Bermuda and was a cofounder of the Merrimack Valley NAACP. I knew from an early age that I was going to help people. I leaned into my perceived strengths and considered teaching. I also have an artistic side and interior decorating was even an option! However, my godmother was a midwife at the time that I was looking at colleges, and I admired her work. Also, I found it common that people would confide in me with some very personal things, including their health and their life challenges. This happened in my neighborhood. This happened on the train. This happened in the library. I knew that I needed to understand that my calling was being able to see and recognize a person's inner self and health struggles that can improve their quality of life and change lives.

Once I answered the call of nursing, I knew I had to get to work. In high school, I inquired about working in a hospital and got a job in the Student Success Jobs program at Brigham and Women's

Hospital. The program is geared for high school students from the city of Boston that are interested in health careers. It is still in existence today and is a fabric of the institution.

Describe Your Admission to a Nursing Program

My admission to nursing was quite traditional. I looked at six different schools, and the program that I chose, Simmons College (now Simmons University), was based on my appreciation of the practice of a few nurse practitioners that I worked with at the time that I was an emergency department unit secretary. I admired their bedside manner. More importantly, I also admired their poise and grace when caring for patients and interacting with colleagues.

Progression and Challenges in the Program

When I went to college, I took my prerequisites, and I was excited to get into the school. However, inorganic chemistry was a challenge for many, as our class went from 135 students to 89 from the fall to spring semester. I ended up taking that class over the summer to boost my GPA so that I could start my nursing core classes. I attended a competitive exam school for a rigorous high school education, which included the classical languages, but it was not science focused. I went to a program and was tutored by nuns on how to take multiple-choice exams. The experience was invaluable. Having been in advanced classes and attending an exam school since the fourth grade helped me understand the competitiveness of school, but nursing school was like none other. Every single exam predicted the outcome of your potential academic and professional career. The pressure was mind-crushing. However, I endured the rigor. I learned. I grew. I persevered. I kept my eye on the prize.

One of the struggles that I had in college overall was that I lived at home my first year. It helped me to understand that I needed to be a part of a community. Not being a resident at school or being involved in activities and clubs that help to round out a college experience actually almost contributed to me leaving or transferring. However, I really enjoyed college, and I found people who really believed in me. Once I moved on campus, I felt like a real college student. In addition to moving on campus with the help of friends, I was able to be involved in the Black Student Organization, as well as start the African American, Latino, Asian, and Native American (ALANA) Student Nursing Association so there was a place and a space for nursing students of color.

In contrast, I noticed that while I was receiving an excellent education, I felt like the billboards that said that my university was inclusive did not match my experience. The cognitive dissonance was experienced not only by me but also some of my student colleagues who had to choose alternative academic plans. As a student, I was furious, and I went to the dean's office asking to meet with her. We had a spirited discussion about academics, access, opportunities, NCLEX pass rates, the Black student experience, and the Black student nursing experience. One of the last things that I had said to her at the time was, "When I come to school, it's not just about me. I have people looking for me to succeed. I have family members looking up to me to see what I'm going to do, which will help them eventually go to college. My degree, yes, it's for me, but it's not about me. I've rested on too many shoulders to come this far and not succeed." The dean started to invite me to meetings that focused on the education gaps within the school of nursing that focused on prerequisite success and NCLEX pass rates. There was a direct correlation between unsuccessful or lower grade prerequisites and not passing the NCLEX on the first attempt. I completed that program with a baccalaureate in nursing with a double minor in biology and Africana studies and passed my NCLEX on the first attempt.

After serving on hospital and unit-based nursing practice councils, I came to understand that I did not just love nursing practice but what drives nurses to care for their patients. To get behind supporting that *why*, I enrolled at Emmanuel College Nursing program and earned a master's degree in nursing leadership and management. To further my education even more, I enrolled in a nursing PhD program to further my learning and expand opportunities for nursing involvement as the healthcare landscape rapidly changes.

Share About Your First Job and Your Career Progression

Little did I know, my advocacy at Simmons helped me to lay the groundwork for the start of the Dotson Bridge and Mentoring Program (Christian et al., 2021). The program focuses on nursing students of color by matching them with mentors and providing additional academic and social supports to ensure their success. Oftentimes, the program is able to have special events or seminars that the entire school of nursing is able to attend. The Dotson program is not just life changing for the students but also for the school. Students feel like they have a place where they can belong, and the nursing program has the most diverse student body compared with other majors in the college. Just in 2020, more than 50% of the freshman class was from a background who didn't identify as White. Simmons and the Dotson Bridge and Mentoring Program have really been intentional about tomorrow's nurses having ethnic-cultural concordance with the patients they serve.

Since the inception of the program, I have served as a mentor in the program and also on the advisory board.

Outside of Simmons, I joined the New England Regional Black Nurses Association (NERBNA) as a student. During my senior year, Simmons and the executive director of the National Black Nurses Association (NBNA) sponsored students to attend the National Black Nurses Association conference. I've never looked back since. In the national and local levels of NERBNA and NBNA, respectively, I was able to learn how to be a young professional nurse and give back to my community, as well as write, speak, and present on national platforms during our annual conferences. NBNA/NERBNA has been my home throughout my academic and professional career. I subsequently joined Sigma Theta Tau as a community leader and continued my volunteer work in various nursing professional organizations as my career progressed. In my senior clinical practicum rotation, I learned to hone my skills on a medical stepdown unit. I quickly realized that I love this population. Upon graduation, I had two offers: one for a new unit and the second on an orthopedic unit. I chose the 31-bed medical stepdown unit. There, I worked hard, grew my practice, and earned a position as a nurse in charge while I was in graduate school. Shortly after completing my master's degree, I earned the position for the inaugural Mairead Hickey Nursing Leadership Fellowship. There, I was able to position and socialize myself as a new nurse leader while understanding the operations and organization of health care overall. Once I completed this program, I had no idea what kind of job I wanted to have because I was completely content with caring for my patients. However, a position for a nurse administrator became available. Then, full circle, I was trained by the very nurse leader who hired me as a unit secretary in the emergency department. I learned how to keep a 793-bed hospital running safely on the night shift. I moved to work evenings and eventually was asked to help build a day role that focused on the throughput of hospital operations but primarily focused on bed flow and patient access to care. After building this role, I became the nurse director for the IV Therapy team and subsequently the Patient Care Associate (CNA) Float Pool. Leading these two teams has been an absolute gift to my personal and professional growth. In addition, it gives me great joy to work with both of these teams to give them a voice for themselves and for the patients that they serve.

Recommendations for Equity in the Future

There is a seat for everyone at the table. Just because another seat is added does not mean another is taken away. Nursing is having critical staffing shortages, and it is necessary that we do an environmental scan of how we procure and grow each other. We must end the "fork in the road" educational path system. Are you a person of color? Do you have a name that is hard to pronounce? Do you have an accent? Do you have limited resources to get into nursing? The educational path should be the same for you as anyone else. Encouraging people to get a job as a CNA at a major facility or enter an ADN program knowing they cannot gain a nursing position in the facility in which they work; not providing financial and academic resources to encourage success; and not giving them the guidance and resources on how to successfully transition to a BSN program

There is a seat for everyone at the table. Just because another seat is added does not mean another is taken away.

perpetuate structural racism. We lose so many talented diverse nurses this way, as they are relegated to nonacute care facilities as a first nursing job. We then penalize their knowledge and skills gap when they finally enter acute care. You cannot say someone is "not a good fit" or "cannot keep up with the pace" when they walked in the door on an unlevel playing field and with a continually moved goal post. For nursing to have a racial/ethnic caregiver–patient concordance, we need to look at high school education (and even earlier) to give students the anticipatory guidance on what is required for nursing school enrollment and retention. Once they receive this guidance, they actually need to be provided with resources to obtain a quality education.

Nursing is a sacred calling, and the profession of tomorrow depends on the profession we construct today. Nursing needs all of us.

If you are already in nursing, no matter the level, my advice is to get involved and stay visible. Show up for your patients. Show up to professional events. Show up for yourself. Find a mentor. What is your contribution to the profession? Are you letting change happen around you, or are you working to influence change? Find the leader within you. Are you an advocate? Are you an ally in fighting racism in nursing? How will you use your privilege to impact positive change? Nursing is a sacred calling, and the profession of tomorrow depends on the profession we construct today. Nursing needs all of us.

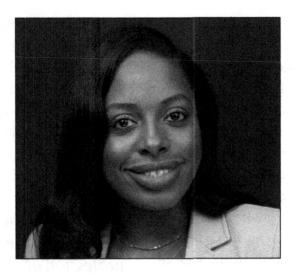

Sasha DuBois, MSN, RN

Sasha DuBois, MSN, RN, is a nurse director at Brigham and Women's Hospital (BWH) in Boston, MA. Invested in nursing education, mentoring, and the development of tomorrow's nurses, she works as a mentor at the Simmons University Dotson Bridge and Mentoring Program. Sasha received her BSN with a minor in Africana studies and biology from Simmons College and an MSN from Emmanuel College in Nursing Leadership and Management. Sasha invests in the progression, visibility, perception, and preservation of the nursing profession. She has served on her hospital Nursing Practice Committees and Magnet initiatives to engage clinical nurses on the importance of Magnet Designation.

Sasha serves as the secretary for the National Black Nurses Association (NBNA) and president of the New England Black Regional Nurses Association and sings in her church's young adult choir. She is also a member of the American Nurses

Association and Association of Nurse Leaders (AONL) and has actively served on various community boards. She is also a mentor for the BWH/Roxbury Community College partnership as well as directs the Brigham and Women's Hospital Neskey Educational Opportunity for PCAs. A Boston native, Sasha DuBois is a highly motivated emerging leader and continues to seek ways to give back to her profession as well as her community.

6

If You Can Count Them, There Aren't Enough

Greg Durkin MEd, RN, NPDA-BC*

Why Did You Choose Nursing as a Career?

Before I begin my story, I want to say that I will be sharing some experiences as examples. These experiences are not presented with the intention of pointing a finger of shame or derision toward any individual or group. They are presented with the intention of illustrating the perspective of an underrepresented member of the nursing community.

I wish I could say that I had a noble commitment to the betterment of mankind, or that my experience as a hospitalized child informed my lifelong journey in nursing. The reality of how I ended up choosing nursing as a career is a lot different and a little bit complicated to describe.

I grew up in Dearborn, MI, in a blue-collar, lower middle-class family. We didn't have what anyone could describe as a surplus of money or things, but what we did have were parents who valued the importance of an education and contributing to community. I was reasonably intelligent, I guess, and it was always assumed I would graduate high school and go to college. We never talked about it in any real way; it was just assumed, even though neither of my parents had been successful in graduating from higher education nor had many of my extended family. In high school, I was doing well in the sciences, and my peers would talk about career options; frequently, healthcare professions would come up. This was the early 80s, so the breadth of options was less obvious to us, and what we talked about was medicine, nursing, or medical technology. I remember taking a career assessment test of some nature, and the results suggested I would be most successful as a "dietitian" despite my fondness for sweets, McDonald's, and Coca-Cola. Clearly, becoming a dietitian was not for me, and I dismissed the entire report.

At this time, my mother, at the age of 40, returned to university to complete a degree she had started nearly 20 years earlier (talk about a commitment to lifelong learning). Neither of my parents nor any of my extended family were in a healthcare profession; I did not have that exposure. During my mother's initial studies, she met and became close friends with a woman named Karen (not her real name) who would soon become a fixture in our house on weekends. Karen was in nursing school, and I watched her study or talk about her clinical experiences, or hear her stories of the struggles and successes, I would regularly find myself thinking, "This looks like something I would like to study and pursue," but I didn't talk about it much. Why? Because this was 1982, and I was a young man who was not quite ready to deal with his sexual orientation (more on that later). As a point of history, a man choosing nursing as a career in 1982 was not exactly encouraged, and it came with a lot of judgment, stereotypes, and jokes. I put it out of my head and started my higher education at a community college, taking advanced math and science courses and thinking maybe I'd work in a lab or, who knows, maybe pursue medicine.

During my first year, I learned in my inorganic chemistry class that I detested lab work. There was nothing less interesting to me than being given a substance called "unknown" and having to figure out what it was. I was much happier with anatomy, biology, and sociology. There ended any vision of medical technology!

In community colleges, you do not find a lot of premed students—at least then you didn't. They were in universities and driven toward getting into med school right from the beginning. Free from influence and opportunities, thoughts of becoming a physician faded from my brain—although, honestly, they were never there very strongly to begin with. In my classes, I was surrounded, however, by many peers who were either already pursuing nursing or planning on going to nursing school. Somewhere toward the end of my first year, I decided to join them. How did I choose nursing? By exposure. By people talking about the benefits of the career, by meeting people committed to education and scientific studies, and by being surrounded by like-minded people who didn't find anything strange about a 19-year-old young man entering into a female-dominated profession; it may not have been normalized in the external world, but it was in that community of learners. It also just happened to be consistent with my family's values about contributing to the betterment of community and society, about ongoing education and learning, and about working toward a profession that would provide stable employment.

Describe Your Admission to a Nursing Program

In the summer between my first and second years of community college, I made the decision to become a nurse. As I said previously, it was always assumed I would go to college, but what I didn't say is that it was also assumed that I would graduate from a university with a bachelor's degree. My parents had strong feelings about the importance of that, so obtaining an associate degree in nursing was never really an option, even though Karen had recently graduated with her ADN and was now employed and happy. Because of my family's finances, going away to university also wasn't really an option—I learned from an early age that opportunities are not equally distributed to communities and groups. In high school, my guidance counselor pushed me to apply to a community college despite graduating in the top 10% of my class, "because your family can't afford it." He then explained my financial options and how, given my scholarship and a PELL grant, my money would go further at a community college. This was irrespective of my potential. I couldn't afford it; that was the end of the discussion. Other students who had similar grades and performance also had this experience and were shepherded to community college. Many of us ended up in the same classes like an extension of high school, while other peers with more resources went away to universities.

> *I learned from an early age that opportunities are not equally distributed to communities and groups.*

I chose to work toward getting accepted to the nursing program at Wayne State University in Detroit, MI. Unbeknownst to me at the time, this was considered one of the best nursing schools. All I knew as a young person was that I could afford the tuition, thanks to financial aid, and I could live at home and commute to class every day. I learned what the prerequisite courses were that I could complete at community college and transfer over, and then set forth completing them. I filled out the application, and I remember having to write an essay about why I wanted to pursue nursing—I don't remember what I wrote, but I do remember that I wrote it by hand on a yellow legal pad! It's important to note that in those days there were no computers, and not everyone had even a type-writer, so it was commonplace to do writing assignments by hand. I can't say for sure, but I have always suspected that the fact that I was a man had a significant impact on my acceptance into nurs-ing school. I was getting solid, if not exceptional, grades in commu-nity college, and I had very little volunteer or personal experience with health care. This is very different from today where potential students need to have a portfolio of experiences to get accepted. What can I say? It was 1984, and things were different. Nursing also didn't have the best reputation in those days, and baccalaure-ate degrees were far from the norm as entry into practice. When I started my first job with my BSN at the Children's Hospital of Michigan in Detroit, I was in the minority, and the nurses with whom I worked referred to us as "bulls&$% nurses."

Progression and Challenges in the Program

I transferred to Wayne State in the fall of 1984, finished prereq-uisites, and then started the 3-year nursing program in January of 1985. I remember my first day in a Nursing 101 class; there were 60 or so of us in a big lecture hall. I was overwhelmed with anxi-ety and excitement to be starting and ready to GO! Because Wayne State is an urban institution, the nursing class was more diverse than any other classes I had been in thus far. It was still overwhelm-ingly White women, but there were 3 or 4 other men and students from several ethnicities. Our professor was a Black woman with an advanced degree. I didn't think anything of it at the time, but looking back on my last 30+ years, it's sort of remarkable, given how our profession continues to struggle with non-White representation, especially in faculty and leadership positions. She was tough and passionate. I can still hear the inflection in her voice. She had a profound influence on me because she was really the first person I encountered who presented nursing as a profession and not a job. My worldview opened, and throughout my studies I encountered instructors, professors, mentors, and coaches, all of whom had at least a master's degree, and most had a doctorate. I had no idea. Karen presented a very different view; she was in a job. Her faculty were not doctorally prepared. She and I would talk about my studies, and she would sometimes be dismissive of the rigor and expectations. "Why do you need to study that?" she would say, "You should have stayed at community college; it's all you need, and you'd be working by now." This was her perception, entry into practice was meeting her needs, and she had no need to consider other options.

Nursing school remains the hardest thing I've ever done in my life. The class work we had was tough. Expectations of us were high. We were told from the beginning that we were being prepared to be leaders and not "just" workers. Heck, I just wanted independence and an income, so I can't say all of that meant a ton to me at the time. My challenges in the program were not about being a man in a female-dominated profession. I have to say that I was accepted as an equal from the first day and never felt less than because I was a man. My biggest challenge was finding a woman to be my patient in the lab for a breast physical exam! I remember being a little self-conscious and unsure how to respond when people asked me about my studies. It used to make me annoyed to be called a "male nurse." We don't refer to Mary as a "female nurse"; we are both nurses. A male colleague shared with me that he had an experience with a female nursing instructor who would regularly say "my token male" when referring to men in her classes. I don't recall anyone saying anything like that to me, but I'm certain that I was similarly tokenized. There was a lot of attention to my being a man as a point of interest; it didn't otherwise benefit or harm me.

What was challenging was the very beginning of awareness that I was not just a man, but a gay man. In the mid-80s, this came with a lot of baggage. "Gay" was associated with deviance, with dysfunction, and with AIDS. I repressed, repressed, repressed and just focused on schoolwork and graduating. It seems strange to talk about it now, when so much of our society has evolved. But at that time, being gay meant being ashamed, and I carried that shame deep inside of me for years.

I developed friendships with several women in my program. Funnily enough, I did not become friends with any of the other men. It's like we were all trying to stay away from each other so we didn't get labeled. I remember one of the guys in my program. He was handsome and wore a lot of plaid—funny what you remember. And I remember other students saying they thought he was gay. It was chatter and gossip and reinforced in me that this was something I did not want to admit to or become. I repressed. I focused on my studies and took a part-time job in retail to help pay for a car and school supplies. I was so busy I didn't have time to think about dating or romance of any type, and this busyness kept my peers from making assumptions about me. It was a protective mechanism, I suppose.

Challenges that I had were mostly similar to challenges everyone else had: keeping up with the volumes of reading assigned to us each week, learning new and complicated pathophysiology, studying for incredibly hard exams, and performing well in clinical placements.

In my first clinical placement, we were sent to a long-term care facility, a nursing home in those days. The focus was not on clinical care, but on developing interpersonal relationships and understanding generational differences. Early in my placement, I was walking down the hall and I had an immediate realization: I belonged. I wanted to be part of this profession, and this was where I was meant to be.

Our subsequent clinical placements were all in hospitals and organizations in Detroit, a diverse city and full of people who were different from the very White city where I grew up. The community I grew up in was made up of people from Anglo-European or Middle Eastern heritage. There were no Black students in my school. There were handfuls of students of other ethnicities, but as I say regularly, "If you can count them, there aren't enough." I remember not even hearing the word "Jewish" until I was 19 or 20; where I grew up was White and Catholic. Obviously, that doesn't represent the totality of experiences, but overall, it was a very homogenous community in terms of race/ethnicity. Being in Detroit presented a new set of challenges for me as a White "heterosexual" man: how to relate to a wide array of patient populations from backgrounds and lifeways that I knew very little about. All I knew was what I had experienced as I grew up. The faculty were mostly great about this, pushing and helping us. My clinical instructor during my psych/mental health rotation was amazing. I had a client who was schizophrenic, and during a conversation with him one day, he made a pass at me during our interaction, saying some fairly explicit things and grabbing my leg. I was still not accepting of my sexuality, so this shook me. I talked to my instructor about it, and she started by laughing, "This is not something I usually hear from my male students!" Then she gave me a lesson in what women have to deal with regularly: unwelcomed advances. She told me what to say, how to set boundaries, and how to respond in a way that was firm but wouldn't escalate the situation. These are skills I would later use in my own life.

I had some real struggles in my OB/GYN rotation. We were based in a city hospital where the majority of patients were not White. One of my patients was a Black teenage girl who had just had a baby. Things were going fine, and we worked well together until she was asking about my schooling, and I told her that after I was done with the shift, I had to write a paper about the experience. Shortly after that, the instructor pulled me aside to talk to me because the patient had refused to let me back in the room. I was shocked—I thought we had gotten along so well. She asked me why I was going to write the *Detroit Free Press* about my experience. I then learned about the power of words and communicating more clearly. The patient had heard, "I am going to write the paper about you." The instructor wasn't pleased with me and my ignorance, but she talked to the patient, and we were able to finish the shift together. A couple of weeks later, we were in the nursery. I was taking care of an infant with mottled black and white skin, next to two Black students who had infants of their own to take care of. "Look, you guys, my baby is mixed," I said. Now, these two students could have reacted in a variety of ways, but I am forever grateful at their grace and gentle teasing. They laughed and asked me what I was talking about. They talked to me about my preconceptions and why I had them and helped me understand that what I said was wrong and offensive. Just then, our instructor came in to see how we were doing, and they shared with her what I had said. My instructor was less understanding. I don't remember what she said, but I remember the look on her face and the tone of her voice. It was assumed that I should not be as ignorant as I was. I didn't finish that rotation with a stellar review.

In my last year of nursing school, my mother had by then graduated with her baccalaureate and was completing a master's degree in educational psychology. For her graduate thesis in 1987, she had done a study about gay men and their relationships with their fathers. This was way before I came to terms with my own sexuality. Her hypothesis was that these relationships were strained. She had a friend escort her into gay bars and recruit men to come talk to her about their experiences. Take a moment and think about a 40-something heterosexual woman in 1987 doing this! It boggles the mind. She had finished her data analysis and was sharing her results with us at home. During lunch at school one day, I had mentioned to some of the other students what my mother had done—even then I knew it was something amazing. To my surprise, these students were super interested and wanted me to share her study and results. The next day, I brought in her manuscript and for the first time in my life had a conversation with others in my peer group who did not view being gay as a point of shame. They were intellectually curious about the study, and there was not a single pejorative word said. This was a turning point for me in starting to accept who I was.

Share About Your First Job and Your Career Progression

In March of 1986, at the completion of my pediatric clinical rotation, I left my retail job and took a position as a student nurse technician on a surgical unit at the Children's Hospital of Michigan in Detroit. I still had a year plus to go in my program, but I consider this my first nursing job. I worked the midnight shift on weekends and went to class during the week. The nurses I worked with were older, skillful, and jaded. They had never worked with a man in nursing before, so I was a curiosity. I was accepted as any other employee for the most part, but was often given patients who were bigger, or challenging, or who "needed some male influence," as they used to say. In the med room, there was a calendar on the wall that featured nearly naked men in the photos. This was my first real experience with objectification, but I didn't say anything. The nearly 2 years I held that position were incredibly fundamental to my growth and socialization into the profession.

I learned how to manage a large patient assignment—it was common to be assigned 12 patients on my shift to care for under the RN's supervision. I learned dressing changes, postoperative care, and how to do rapid assessments. I learned how to chart effectively and how to relate to the interprofessional team. These experiences helped me excel in the remainder of the nursing program. I also learned that nursing had an image problem; the popular media was full of images of the sexy nurse or the gay "male nurse." I was constantly assumed to be gay (even though I still had not come out at this point and was actively in denial). Whenever I talked to people about my job, I found myself having to defend what I was doing and protest that I WAS NOT GAY. "Are you going to go back to med school?" That was a question I got way more times than I could count. A man didn't belong here—my nursing colleagues never said that, but everyone else in my life did. I had no role models; there were no men in nursing leadership positions that I remember. We were all staff nurses and mostly in the OR or ICU. There were very few of us on a medical or surgical unit. The few men I did work with went out of their way to show that they were heterosexual—constantly talking about girlfriends, wives, or children. Everything seemed to be filtered through the heterosexual experience, and I had no one to talk to. In retrospect, it was incredibly oppressive to be in that environment. I wonder how my life would have been different had there been a more inclusive culture at the time.

Challenges

In January 1988, I took a position on the same unit as a new graduate RN. Even though I had nearly 2 years of experience on the unit, there were still challenges with role transition and reality shock, but I believe that mostly these were the same as what my female colleagues were experiencing. I continued to work on that unit until 1995.

Sometime in 1989, I was made the permanent afternoon shift charge nurse. Sort of incredible to think that after a bit over one year of professional nursing, I was being given this responsibility. The decision had more to do with being incredibly short-staffed and less to do with my gender or skill. I developed a friendship with the afternoon charge nurse on a neighboring unit; she had a little more experience than I did and was a source of support. I wouldn't call her a mentor, but there may have been aspects of that to our relationship. One afternoon she asked to talk to me; she was visibly upset. One of her patient's parents had complained to management that she had been racially offensive toward them. She was White, and the patient and family were Black. Interestingly, even in an urban hospital at that time, most of the nursing staff were White women, while most of the patients were people of color. She was upset because she didn't see herself as being racist in any way. She said to me, "Before this conversation, I don't believe I ever saw the color of my patients, and now it's all I see. I feel like I am changed and only think about what I'm saying and am I treating them differently." She didn't see this as growth; she saw it as a backward step. It made me reflect on my own behavior.

Fast-forward to the spring of 1992. I was thinking about going back to school to get a master's degree but also seriously struggling with coming out. Nurse colleagues constantly were trying to fix me up with someone (always female) and pressuring me to date. To my knowledge, no one at work suspected that I might in fact be gay. In retrospect, I laugh at this: How could they NOT know? I was overweight at that time and started an unhealthy diet and exercise program; I lost 50 pounds in 4 months. I got much attention for the weight loss, most of it positive, one experience less so.

In the late spring of 1992, I got a call from the director of nursing. She wanted to see me. I had been functioning as cochair of a new "shared governance" effort, staff nurse council, so I expected the meeting would be about that. I sat down in her office, and she looked me in the eye and said, "Greg, I have to ask you something. (pause) Are you sick?"

"No, no," I responded, "I have been on a diet and needed to lose this weight." What I didn't say was that the weight loss also gave me confidence to finally come out to myself and some very close friends who I did not work with. It was still a secret at work. In the late 80s and early 90s, HIV and AIDS were in full-blown social hysteria. It was on the news, in public service announcements, in entertainment. And in those days, asking someone "Are you sick?" was code for "Do you have HIV/AIDS?" I was very aware that this was her connotation, and I was mortified. It wasn't uncommon to lose your job, especially at a hospital. That conversation is something I have never forgotten: how it made me feel, how it reinforced to me that I was "bad," that being gay was something to be ashamed of and hide from.

But I had come out and was starting to date. I was living a double life, presenting myself as straight at work and making up excuses to my nursing colleagues about why I didn't need a date for a coworker's wedding, trying to navigate being gay in the time of HIV/AIDS in my personal life—and still not coming out to my family. I finally did that over the winter of 1992 and was feeling more confident as a full adult human. I got accepted to the School of Education at Wayne State in the spring of 1993—there was no such thing as an MSN in nursing education then, so I went to Education. In the late spring, I went to the Gay and Lesbian March in Washington, DC. This was a transformative experience. I was surrounded by hundreds of thousands of out and proud people. It was affirming and shook off years of isolation. I came home from that and called a local gay and lesbian organization called Affirmations and started to do volunteer work (in between working and going to grad school and trying to date—how did I ever find the energy?). I was dating, and slowly coming out to people at work. It was painful and difficult, and some of my best friends from nursing school stopped talking to me. "I'm glad you have people who support you, but I cannot," one friend told me. She was from an ethnic minority and in a relationship with a man from a different ethnic minority, so no stranger to prejudice, and she couldn't accept me. Another nurse colleague told me, "I feel like you are a different person, and I don't know you anymore." Another friend thought I was going to ask her to move from being friends to being romantic partners. Compare this with the current environment in which lesbian, gay, bisexual, trans, questioning, intersex, asexual, plus (LGBTQIA+) persons in many areas have a vastly different experience. The advent of support networks in middle and high schools, greater visibility, and even same-sex marriage have improved things for many, but far from all, LGBTQIA+ people.

Later that year, the director of Affirmations called me. There was a journalist from the *Detroit Free Press* who wanted to write an article about someone who was impacted by the March on Washington, and he recommended me. (Fun fact, that journalist was Frank Bruni, who has gone on to have a long career at the *New York Times*.) I was interviewed and had my picture taken, and an article appeared in the newspaper in the human-interest section, sort of buried. I figured no one would see it, and that would be that.

The day after the article appeared, I came into the hospital via an employee entrance. Right outside the security office was a bulletin board highlighting notable employees. On that board was the article and my picture. I had just come out to every single employee of my hospital as well as the entire Detroit metropolitan area. The bulletin board was positive and even complimentary, but I was panicked. I was worried about what was going to happen when I got up to the floor—by this point in my career I had been promoted to staff development instructor, so was seen as a leader (my nursing school faculty were right). I had several colleagues already separate from me. And a nurse on another floor (also a gay man) had recently stopped working because he was HIV positive, and the shame that was going around about that was significant. For additional context about the attitudes of the time, I attended my 10-year high school reunion and sat at a table with several peers who were discussing the recent death of a very popular student from our graduating class. He had died of AIDS, and the opinion at the table was adamant that he had caught it by injecting intravenous drugs, there was no way he could have been gay. In their hierarchy, being an IV drug addict was better, and more understandable, than being gay. I was shaking as I walked to the elevator.

To my surprise, I was met with business as usual. Some staff had seen the article and offered their support and friendship. Other staff said nothing, and we kept on doing our work. I was relieved, but the fear of what might happen was real—would I lose my friends? Would I lose my job? Can you be a gay man and work at a children's hospital? There was a lot of mythology at the time that gay men were pedophiles, so it was a reasonable fear. I continued to be nervous until the article disappeared and was replaced by some newer news. One afternoon, an attending physician approached me and asked to talk to me. This particular physician had a lot of stereotypical behaviors of an effeminate gay man. I had heard many staff gossip and talk about him derogatorily over the years. He brought me over to an alcove by the service elevators. I had no idea what he would want to say to me because his specialty was not one that we saw much of on my unit. He raised his arm and pointed at my face, and said in a firm but hushed tones, "You need to shut up."

"What?" I replied.

"You need to stop talking to people about being gay. If you keep being open about this, it will RUIN your career and your future. You will lose your job."

He proceeded to quickly tell me that he knew this from experience as he was a gay man and no one knew. He had to hide it or else he would have been let go a long time ago. Then he wished me good luck and walked away and never said another word to me again.

Opportunities

During my staff nurse experience, there was a new movement blossoming to promote men in nursing. I can't recall for sure, but I think there was even a start-up journal about it. Suddenly we were seeing more male nursing students and hiring more men as staff nurses. I tried to organize the men in the hospital to create a collective voice but was unsuccessful. I'm not sure why. This was an opportunity then, and it is an opportunity to this day.

I was also very aware of the image problem that the nursing profession had, and being proud of my work wasn't enough. I was interested in seeing that image change and for nurses to get the respect they/we deserved. Times were changing, and old school behaviors like nurses giving up their seats in the charting room so that the physicians could sit were no longer happening. When I was a new graduate, I had an interaction with the chief resident of surgery. He had written orders for a patient on our unit that didn't seem exactly right to me. He was rounding, and I took the opportunity to speak with him. I told him that I didn't think one of the orders was appropriate for the patient, to which he responded, "Sir, you don't get paid to think. You get paid to follow orders." This coming from a man who was no more than 2 years older than me. And interestingly, I was always referred to as "sir," while my female colleagues were always referred to by their first names. We had an image problem.

I asked and was given approval to start a new committee called the Image of Nursing at Children's Hospital (INCH). We were a very grassroots group who talked about problems we had experienced or observed and explored ways we could try to change our image. We created a newsletter; there had not been one just for nurses at that time. The newsletter highlighted improvements nurses made, accomplishments, and even some humor. It was amateur hour, but the intention was sincere. We even held a fashion show one year to encourage nurses to dress more professionally.

In the mid-90s, I had met a nurse, Carol (not her real name). After a class I had taught where I had been open about being gay, she came up to me and identified herself as lesbian. This was the first person I had met there who was open about who they were and not ashamed of it. She and I talked about our experiences, about feeling isolated and alone, and about how we both had a desire to create change. Over several conversations, we decided we should try to create a support network of other gay and lesbian employees. It is important to note that at that time, the perspective was fairly myopic to just gay and lesbians and not inclusive of the full continuum of LGBTQIA+ as is more common today. Again, the fear returned. Would we be allowed to do this? Would we get in trouble? Despite the progress being made in society and in ourselves, we still felt the need to hide; we still had some sliver of shame. We made an appointment with the CNO to talk about our idea. I can't say for sure, but I'm pretty confident our voices were shaking as we explained our goal of creating a support network. The CNO was a bit taken by surprise by our request for permission to start such a group, and she admitted to not fully understanding why it was necessary. She gave cautious approval and suggested we try to gather outside the hospital; we shouldn't use hospital property to meet. We support you, but we don't really support you, in essence.

Carol and I were okay with this idea. We were people of our time and had bought into the idea that this might be okay but needed to be hidden. We created a simple flier and nervously posted it in some staff areas. We would meet in the cafeteria of a neighboring hospital down the street. We sat in that cafeteria a couple of times with a sign with just a pink triangle on it—this is symbology that has been associated with being gay from the time of the Holocaust, when gay people were given a pink triangle patch to wear in the concentration camps. I think we had maybe two other people ever come to join us. They were also afraid to let anyone know of their sexuality and were resistant to anything more public or any other action. Needless to say, this effort did not last. Compare this to today's environment in which LGBTQIA+ support groups are in many hospitals and healthcare organizations and even march in pride parades, fully supported.

Milestones

There were several milestones I experienced in my early years in nursing. Being one of a small number of men in my nursing school and being fully accepted was significant. The faculty and students didn't pay attention to my gender. I was just another student. When I was a staff nurse, I became aware of how I was treated a little differently than my female colleagues. Physicians would refer to me sort of respectfully as "sir," while they were "Nancy," or "Sue." I also noticed that their tone was different and that I was listened to more. I used that, in a way, to help me advance. When I was made permanent afternoon charge nurse, that helped others see me as a leader. I was picked out to become one of the first cochairs of a newly formed thing called Staff Nurse Council, and that experience gave me visibility.

For the first time for many of my colleagues, they were working next to and with an openly gay person and forced to rethink their assumptions.

Coming out in a public way was another huge milestone. For the first time for many of my colleagues, they were working next to and with an openly gay person and forced to rethink their assumptions. Forming a committee to address the image of nursing helped me to reinforce our deserving of respect, and it also empowered others. Attempting to start a gay and lesbian support network helped me to bury the shame and move forward to be more open about my sexuality, to advocate on behalf of our needs and experiences, and even to fall in love. Being promoted to staff development instructor in 1990 was the most significant milestone. I was then the only man in a leadership role in the hospital (to the best of my memory), and I was now also a visible gay man in a decision-making capacity. This role transition also helped me discover my true calling: nursing professional development, a specialty practice which I have embraced for the past 30 plus years.

Current Role

I am currently the director of clinical education and informatics at Boston Children's Hospital. My team is centralized and responsible for all throughputs in the nursing professional development practice model: orientation/onboarding, competency management, role development, collaborative practice, education, and EBP/QI/Research. In addition to my work responsibilities, I have several side activities. I have been an editorial board member for the *Journal for Nurses in Professional Development* for over a decade. I have published articles on web-based education, professional posters, competency management, self-advocacy, and preceptor support. I am involved in several activities with the Association for Nursing Professional Development (ANPD), including as a faculty member for the Certification Preparation Review Course, the Board of Directors Nominating Committee, and the Scope and Standards revision working group, and I have

> *I am one of a very small number of men and one of the few openly gay (or LGBTQIA+) persons at the table.*

participated in several publications. I have also presented numerous times at ANPD conventions. In all of those activities, I am one of a very small number of men and one of the few openly gay (or LGBTQIA+) persons at the table.

Challenges

There remain many challenges to equity, diversity, inclusion, and belonging in our profession. Specific to my place in the specialty practice of nursing professional development and as leader, there continues to be an absence of men. While our numbers have grown since 1986, at my organization, I am one of a handful of men in a formal leadership position. At my organization there are well over 100 nurses in formal leadership roles, yet there are just over 10 men in these roles. I am positive there are more LGBTQIA+ individuals in these roles, but I can name less than five who have made that open knowledge. Every individual makes their own decision about how open to be. Is the environment supportive? Is there potential for backlash? Is it seen as unimportant? Throughout my 35 years in nursing, there has been an absence of male role models or peer support in the organizations for which I have worked. I have worked in three different hospitals, two universities, and a public health organization. Almost always, when I am in a meeting, or a workshop, or any group really, I look around and am the only man in the room, and just as often the only openly gay person in the room. This has a cumulative

> *Throughout my 35 years in nursing, there has been an absence of male role models or peer support in the organizations for which I have worked.*

effect of being supremely isolating. I used to shrug it off and say humorously that in nursing I was a prejudice double coupon.

In the mid-1990s, I interviewed for a position at a public health organization in Philadelphia, PA. During my interview, the executive director sat across from me and said that she really liked me and what I could bring to the organization. She then said she was concerned about hiring me: "You have two liabilities for me that I am not sure how to address. You are a man. And you are White. I already have too many White people working here, and I've never hired a man before for this work." This was an organization that worked primarily with underserved, low-income populations of color, and the client base was nearly exclusively pregnant women or women with small children at home. While the question undoubtedly raises eyebrows, I understood where she was coming from. I must have answered satisfactorily because I was hired and worked there very happily for nearly 5 years.

> **Individuals who are less represented have a harder time accessing opportunities.**

I moved to Boston in the summer of 2002 and started working at Boston Children's Hospital later that year. Again, I was in a role in which I was the only man in the department and the only openly gay person on my team. Management opportunities presented themselves over the years, but my role stayed the same while I watched several junior staff leap over me into them. I was qualified, a high performer, and would have welcomed the chance. What remains to be true in my experience is that individuals who are less represented have a harder time accessing opportunities.

I remember one (rare) time at an organization when I was offered a management role in my department. When I accepted, my boss at the time said to me, "You need to find a mentor." There was no offer of assistance in finding such a person in the organization, and when I asked for suggestions, my boss replied, "I'm not sure there is anyone in the organization who will meet your needs, you are going to have to look outside." Contrast this with other female managers who had been recently promoted: They were given names of other leaders who could function as a mentor, and their bosses ensured that the mentoring relationships were formed. Consequently, I have never had a long-term formal mentoring relationship. This is not specific to my current workplace; I have never had such a relationship in 35 years. Sure, there have been people (all women) I have tapped into for help, support, coaching, or informal mentoring. All of those relationships were, and continue to be, effective, but I have never had access to a man in nursing and have never had a member of the LGBTQIA+ community to serve this purpose. Additionally, female colleagues who were similarly promoted were encouraged to join nursing leadership organizations, attend leadership conferences, and gain skills. I was never offered or encouraged to take advantage of these things, and I cannot say what the rationale was; I just know that I was treated differently. Having a male and/or LGBTQIA+ mentor would have helped me address challenges in a way that heterosexual women cannot. Many times throughout my career it would have been helpful to have someone like that to help me navigate being a man in a female-dominant profession or to help me deal with questions and ignorance of LGBTQIA+ experiences.

I identify as a cisgender, White, gay man. This, in and of itself, is not remarkable. Over the past decade, the emergence of a broader array of sexual orientations and the now more commonplace LGBTQIA+ collective has been a challenge. Early in my career, I felt a responsibility to represent the gay male experience. I felt pressure to be "normal" and "fit in" and be part of the broader society. This had the effect of isolating my full identity and prevented me from self-actualization. I would talk in nonspecific terms about who I lived with or what I do. I would edit what I said and treat every new interaction with trepidation. Is this person "safe"? Can I share my whole self, or will I be treated differently? Will they understand my life and my cultural norms, and will they be accepting? Many LGBTQIA+ people treat every new interaction with a complex algorithm to determine what they can or cannot say. This happens at work, at school, in hotels, in taxicabs, everywhere.

As the understanding and evolution of the gay experience to be more inclusive of the LGBTQIA+ spectrum has happened, I had my own personal challenges. What does this broader representation mean, and where is my place in it? I had my own evolution to do. While I was comfortable in my identity as a cisgender, White, gay man, I was less comfortable in being part of this broader continuum of identity and experience. I recognize that there are similar challenges for the dominant workforce.

At one point in the recent past, we were beginning an effort to collect sexual orientation and gender identity from our patients to help us provide more equitable care. Being involved in the educational effort around this, I was asked to present to the entire nursing leadership team. At the conclusion of the presentation, one of the nurse managers asked, "Greg, why do we need to ask these questions? Why do we need to care about this?" In front of the entire group, I explained how knowing who our patients are helps us to see the entire person, not just the disease or injury. I then explained how gay people spend their entire lives navigating the hesitance and attitudes of heterosexual people. "I have to completely isolate my existence," I said. "I have a gay doctor, a gay dentist, a gay pharmacist, a gay lawyer, a gay realtor. I plan vacations in gay-accepting locations. I worry about reactions to me in taxicabs, at hotels, and in stores. I spend my entire life tippy-toeing around straight America's sensitivities, and it's time for that to stop. I shouldn't have to hide and neither should our patients." This response was met with gratitude and approval by several of my leadership colleagues. But it was extraordinarily difficult for me because here I was again expected to translate my existence in this world for other people, and to represent all of the LGBTQIA+ experience. It's worth noting that there were a couple other openly LGBTQIA+ leaders in the room and not one of them said anything out loud to back me up. I can't say why that was; it could have been a matter of group dynamics, it may have been an unwillingness to be out, or it may have just been a matter of timing. I received private texts or emails of support but would have really appreciated vocal and verbal support in the moment. There I was, alone again.

My current workplace started a support network several years ago called GLBT and Friends. I started attending with enthusiasm. This was what I had envisioned all those years ago in Detroit and here I was, working for a hospital that was eager to have this inclusion. This is marvelous, I thought! I started attending monthly meetings, where a couple dozen of us would sit in a circle and talk about our experiences, both good and bad. During these meetings, it was very common to start with introductions. We would go around the room and talk about how we identify and what our lives were like. Person after person would say something like, "Hi, I'm Mary, and I'm a lesbian. I have been married to my wife for 10 years, and we have two children." One after another would present this sort of narrative, in a very heteronormative way, one of marriage, children, pets, and a house in the suburbs. This was not my experience. I was not married and didn't want to be. I do not have children and don't want to be a parent. I live in the city and partake in nightlife and travel and have a wide circle of friends with all sorts of existences. At the time, I felt very much like my own "community" had expectations of representation, of how we were supposed to live. Not a single person in those meetings presented a life anything near what I had. Even other gay men in the room who I had interacted with outside of work presented themselves differently and whitewashed their lives. I stopped attending the meetings after a couple months. I wanted a community where all felt like they belonged, where we could talk openly about our different lives, but this group felt very homogenous in a way.

Early in my employment at Boston Children's, I attended a fundraiser for a health center that serves a majority LGBTQIA+ population. It was a costume party, and the effort that participants put forth to express themselves and have some silly fun was enormous. It was common for men to dress in various states of drag or subversive takes on popular culture. I had some (heterosexual) friends at work and told them about the event. They expressed interest in seeing some of my photos. We were working in cubicles, and I pulled up some pictures on a computer. Two colleagues were looking over my shoulder, and we laughed and talked about the joy on participants' faces. Another nurse leader colleague overheard our joviality and came over to see what was going on. She looked at the screen and said, "Who are all these FREAKS?" I shut down the photo display and ended the sharing. This had a chilling effect on me. It would be years before I shared something personal about my life with anyone at work. I wasn't "representing" the community to a level that others expected, apparently, and her judgmental response angered me. Meanwhile, my all female, heterosexual colleagues would freely talk about their husbands, their children, their weddings, on and on. It was, and continues to be, isolating, even in an organization that passes out gay pride rainbow lanyards to all new employees at hospital orientation. It is fascinating to compare this to current times, when *RuPaul's Drag Race* is practically normalized in the broader culture and even wins Emmy Awards without the word "freak" ever being used. Progress has been made, but barely a day goes by when there isn't another news item somewhere about how being LGBTQIA+ is somehow destroying the fabric of society. You have to be pretty thick-skinned to face that every day of your life and keep going.

In an effort to address a practice gap, I was leading a team to design some new leadership education. Each member of the team had content they were responsible for developing, and they had to assess the current scholarly and popular literature. One of the participants pulled up her resources on a big screen in the conference room in front of me and several other staff. The resource she was using was a religious organization which created a set of leadership tools that she thought were effective. On the sidebar of the website was some advertising. One of the advertisements was for a book that was about the downfall of American culture being due to the presence of homosexuality in America. I, of course, do not know if that is what she believed, but the fact that she felt comfortable showing such a thing in front of me and the team was stunning. Having all nursing work be filtered through the lens of cisgendered, White, heterosexual women is, and continues to be, a challenge.

Despite this, I still find myself regularly called upon to explain my life and what it means to be gay. I am asked to help other people learn about my experience when I advocate for myself/others or confront others about something insensitive. Even though I am not bisexual, lesbian, trans, intersex, questioning, or otherwise, I am expected to know what it means to be all of those things and explain the experience. I will say it again, in nursing, all of life is filtered through the lens of a cisgender, White, heterosexual woman because that is who the dominant workforce is, that is who holds positions of power.

I received a call from a man who needed some help with his educational records. There was an error, and he wanted to see if I could correct it. I looked him up by his last name in the learning management system. When I looked over the list of names, I could not find him. "I don't see a Mark in the database," I told him (not his real name). "Oh, try looking for Elizabeth, that's my birth name." I found the record and made the correction, and he and I talked about his experience. Our systems did not allow him to have his name displayed correctly. His payroll, his employment records, even his ID badge had "Elizabeth" on it, requiring him to explain his transition to everyone he encountered. He was not bothered by it, but I was outraged. No one has ever asked me to talk about my gender identity. I approached the director of our human resources function and shared this story. She was similarly upset by it and vowed to figure out a way to make change. That was great, but I was left with questions: Why did this never occur to you or anyone until I brought it up? Why were his concerns, as a non-leadership employee, not addressed until now? Why was it up to me, a non-trans man, to represent his experience? Why wasn't his experience acknowledged and addressed in a timelier way?

Opportunities

Let me be clear, I enjoy working for my hospital and am proud of my organization. Even though I presented some examples of less than positive interactions, I have found tremendous progress in representation and inclusion of men and LGBTQIA+ staff in nursing. Things I never thought were possible 30 years ago are almost commonplace and represent several opportunities for the future of nursing. Additionally, the emergence of the importance of equity, diversity, inclusion, and belonging in all aspects of public, private, and organizational life has had a profound effect on the beginnings of real and lasting change.

The emergence of LGBTQIA+ groups in organizations is a powerful force for such change. My organization has an advisory group, support networks, and public displays of support. We give out pride lanyards to new employees, we have an annual LGBTQIA+ award, we hold pride events, we participate in our city's pride parade, and we have pride and trans pride flag raisings in front of the hospital each June. We have been working to ensure that our medical records accurately represent the sex and gender identities of our patients. The use of taglines in emails and web calls to declare preferred pronouns has become commonplace.

Over my career span, I have definitely observed an increase in the number of men in nursing and in nursing leadership positions. When I started as a unit educator in Detroit, I was the only man in a leadership role at my hospital. Flash-forward to the current day, and there are many others, including one who reports to me. There is still a gap, though, and more effort needs to be made. As a counterpoint, while writing this chapter, a genderqueer colleague presented to me a different narrative. In her perspective, men had an advantage due to embedded patriarchy. She had witnessed men being moved into leadership positions more quickly and in greater numbers in proportion to the number of men in the profession, and once in those positions, she observed them being treated differently and being able to enact their agendas more readily. Relative to the number of women in the profession, there were fewer of them in leadership, proportionally, in her view. Upon reflection, it is true that I was moved into my first leadership role very quickly. However, there were also two other women similarly moved into those positions at the same time as I was, and we all had the same amount of experience. Additionally, I have been working at my current organization for nearly 20 years, and it took almost 15 years for me to be moved into formal leadership. So my experience doesn't completely match her impression. It is provocative, however, to think about this in the greater professional cohort: Is there truth to what she said?

Similar to the number of men and openly LGBTQIA+ individuals, there continues to exist an opportunity to increase the number of Black and Indigenous people of color as well as historically excluded communities in nursing and leadership positions.

Similar to the number of men and openly LGBTQIA+ individuals, there continues to exist an opportunity to increase the number of Black and Indigenous people of color as well as historically excluded communities in nursing and leadership positions. These folks are underrepresented in a significant way, though again, progress has been made. I can count on two hands the number of these folks in formal leadership roles in all of the places I have worked, and none are in executive nursing leadership roles. If you can count them, there aren't enough.

One of the most significant opportunities to influence change is for LGBTQIA+ people to live openly and honestly and not shy away from sharing our lives. There is still some taboo and discomfort. I shouldn't feel discomfort talking about my biological as well as chosen families, just the same as how heterosexual, cisgender folks have no boundaries when talking about their spouses, children, and lives. My goodness, the number of times I have had to endure talk about my heterosexual colleagues' sex lives is immeasurable! (Please stop doing that.) It is imperative for LGBTQIA+ nurses to demand equal treatment and respect. And it is imperative for heterosexual, cisgender nurses to respond to us respectfully with acceptance.

Your Recommendations for Equity in the Future

As we continue our path to more equity in nursing, I have several recommendations for the future. First, nurses in the dominant culture (e.g., White, heterosexual) need to take the initiative to learn and grow and not just wait to be taught. "I'm here to learn," is no longer an appropriate response. Feeling sorry but not taking the blame, denial of intentionality, and displays of tears are weapons that function to take the issues off the table.

Next, we need to promote the understanding of intersectionality. I'm not just White. I'm not just a man. I'm not just a nurse. I'm not just cisgender. I'm not just gay. I am all of these things and more, and every one of us is a composite of primary and secondary characteristics that inform, influence, and direct our lives. Further, it includes the experiences we have had, our influences, our income level, and our

> *Every one of us is a composite of primary and secondary characteristics that inform, influence, and direct our lives.*

beliefs. Viewing each person as a fully realized adult is fundamental to increasing equity, diversity, inclusion, and belonging.

Organizations need to do more than take performative action when it comes to concerns of equity. It's fantastic for our organizations to hang a pride flag or participate in a pride march, but are HR and employment policies truly supportive? Are all aspects of LGBTQIA+ life equally supported and valued? Support needs to be more than a lanyard or words. Are policies in place to treat LGBTQIA+ patients and family members the same as heterosexual ones? Are HR systems enabled to refer to people by preferred names or pronouns? Is there an organization-wide mandate to participate in continuing education? In my organization, I am proud to say we are a leader in health equity for LGBTQIA+ folks. Before we achieve this designation, we need to demonstrate a commitment to continuing education on these issues. Unfortunately, the burden of participation in this education seems to fall disproportionately on LGBTQIA+ staff. We also offer a regular "safe zone" education session for nursing staff, but this is considered optional and not offered in the same frequency for all other employees. Additional questions: Who are we doing business with? Who do we take money from? Are those groups and organizations supportive of inclusiveness? It is all too easy to find countless organizations and corporations who profess a commitment to LGBTQIA+ issues but who then donate money to other individuals and groups who are actively working against those very same issues. We see this hypocrisy, and it erodes confidence and trust.

Additionally, nursing leaders need to actively seek out, mentor, and support LGBTQIA+ individuals and men into employment. They need to create systems and structures to help them advance in their careers so we increase their numbers in leadership positions. Organizations cannot wait for an applicant to appear at their door.

They need to go outside and recruit such individuals to come work for them.

And finally, each of us in the LGBTQIA+ community needs to be open and honest in our visibility and expect acceptance from colleagues. My personal and professional journey has been enabled by people who came before me and demanded inclusion. And then by people who stood beside me when I demanded it. Over the last 3 decades, the view of LGBTQIA+ people has progressed in significant ways. When I was coming out, being gay was looked at with derision and fear, both inside and outside my community. Today, LGBTQIA+ support is increasing everywhere; there are affinity groups in organizations, inclusion in organizational diversity operations, presence of benefits for same-sex partners/spouses, and an increase in positive representation of our lives. In concert with this authentic living, our nursing departments and healthcare organizations need to create cultures in which nonacceptance is not okay.

I am so thankful I chose nursing as my profession, and that nursing professional development found me. I have had a rich career and have impacted, and been impacted by, so many people of all kinds of lifeways and perspectives. Being a gay man in nursing has limited me in some ways, but it hasn't held me back. I continue to engage, enrich, and grow, and it is my belief that nursing can and must do the same so that every single nurse feels they are treated equitably, respected for their diversity, and included.

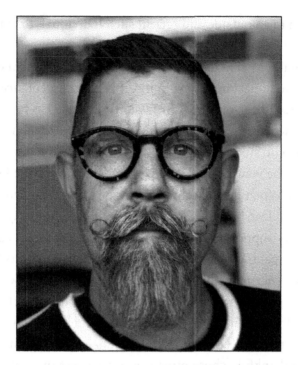

Greg Durkin, MEd, RN, NPDA-BC®

Greg Durkin holds the titles of director of clinical education and informatics and associate director for interprofessional education of the BCH Academy for Teaching and Educational Scholarship and Innovation at Boston Children's Hospital, where he was the recipient of the 2018 Nursing Leadership Award. He has been in the field of professional development since 1990, working in tertiary care, academic, and community health settings. Greg is on the editorial board for the *Journal for Nurses in Professional Development* (*JNPD*) and has published articles on development of web-based courses, orientation evaluation, and competencies. An accomplished speaker, Greg has presented at countless regional and local associations and organizations on diverse topics such as needs assessment, cultural awareness, having a questioning attitude, competency, professional joy, and teamwork. Greg is a past recipient of the ANPD Excellence in Professional Development Educator/Facilitator Practice Award, is a coauthor to the *Certification Preparation Study Guide*, was a section editor for the fifth edition of ANPD's *Core Curriculum for Nursing Professional Development*, and participated in the revision of the *NPD Scope and Standards of Practice*.

7

Transforming Nursing From the Old Guard to the Future

Ernest Grant, PhD, RN, FAAN

I guess I should start this story out by describing how I came to be a nurse. When I was in high school, nursing was the furthest thing from my mind! When I started considering a career, I decided that I wanted to be an anesthesiologist—and drive a 1968 lime green Mercury Cougar with a red leather interior. However, growing up as the youngest of seven children and a widowed mom, I knew that there was probably no money available for me to go to college, let alone medical school. I remember talking with my guidance counselor about my career choice. He stated that I definitely had the grades to get into medical school and that I could probably get some scholarships that would support me through undergraduate school, but the problem may be finding funds or scholarships to pay for medical school. He suggested that I look at nursing as a career. I could become a CRNA, and if I still wanted to go to medical school and become an anesthesiologist, I could work my way through med school as a CRNA making more money than I would as a staff nurse. Then he suggested that I may not like nursing, so he suggested that I take the one-year LPN Course at A-B Technical Institute (now Asheville-Buncombe Technical Community College), and if I liked nursing, I could apply to the ADN program upon completion of the LPN course. About 3 months into the LPN course, I totally forgot about medical school. I realized that nursing was my calling, and I knew that I wanted to achieve my BSN so that I could do more for my patients than the practice restrictions that were placed on my position as an LPN. I very much enjoyed being an LPN, but mostly that role involved doing patient care, and about 90% of the time I worked, I was the medication nurse for the floor that I staffed. I wanted to be an advocate for those in my care. Upon completion of the LPN course, I immediately started taking college courses toward my BSN. I completed my BSN in 1985, graduating from North Carolina Central University (NCCU). After about 5 years with my BSN, I still saw and thought that I could advocate more on behalf of the profession and my patients by achieving my MSN. I completed my MSN in 1993, and 25 years later went back to school and completed my PhD. The time in between the MSN and PhD were very busy years

Being a Black man (perhaps I should qualify that by saying a 6'6" Black man) in a female-dominated profession was a rarity in the late 70s and early 80s.

doing what I loved—advocating for the patients and the profession. I got very busy within the North Carolina Nurses Association (NCNA) and the American Nurses Association (ANA), serving on several committees and boards.

I have faced many challenges during my nursing career. These have ranged from being a Black man in a female-dominated profession to having my qualifications questioned and being told that I was over- or underqualified for certain positions. I shall explain each one of those statements.

Being a Black man (perhaps I should qualify that by saying a 6'6"
Black man) in a female-dominated profession was a rarity in the
late 70s and early 80s. I realized immediately the impression that
I made whenever I would walk the halls of my unit. Being the size
that I was, I could be viewed as being very threatening. However, as
an LPN or even later as an RN, I had to fight to let my female colleagues know that I was their equal and not a muscleman available
to do their heavy lifting. If I wasn't assigned the heavy patients or
all male patients, I frequently would be asked to help lift that heavy
patient in room 405 into a chair or insert a catheter in a young male
patient because my female colleague felt uncomfortable doing
such a procedure. It wasn't that I minded helping my colleagues,
but I also needed to remind them that I was not an orderly. I would
defend my qualifications by stating something like, "I don't mind
helping you lift that patient or inserting that foley, but tell me, what
would you do if I wasn't here today?" In other words, I was making
them think that yes, I'm a team player, but I also am your colleague
with the same initials after my name that you have. You and I took
the exact same courses, and we are both qualified to do the same
job. You asking me to do something that you are very capable of
doing yourself just because I am a male is insulting and unprofessional. They finally got the message after a few times of pointing
that out. I would advise any male going into the nursing profession
to not let yourself be used as an orderly. Stand up for yourself! You
shouldn't have to earn the respect of your colleagues just because
of your gender or the color of your skin.

Regarding having my qualifications questioned, that has happened on so many different occasions and in so many different
settings. I think the first clue that I was having my qualifications
brought into question was around graduation from my BSN program. When colleagues ask you, "What school did you graduate

from?" as if that is going to determine whether or not you are a good nurse, it is insulting, prejudicial, and unprofessional. It shouldn't matter what school an individual graduated from, what matters is that they passed the NCLEX exam which proves that they have met the minimum standard to bear the initials "RN" after their name. To me, the next important factor depends upon whether a seasoned RN takes that individual under their wing and mentors that new nurse. I have seen nurses who have graduated from some of the top schools in the country struggle because they had difficulty applying theory into practice. They were great at understanding concepts and theory, but when it came to actual hands-on practice, there was a roadblock. I firmly believe that it takes all of us working together to mold and mentor each other so that we can all be the best nurse we can be to advocate for our patients and our profession.

I can recall another time in which my qualifications were called into question. I remember applying for a mid-level management position (assistant nurse manager) and being told that I did not have the qualifications for the job. I knew this was a lie because at that time, I had been an RN for 7 years, had obtained a master's degree (the job description stated a BSN degree or higher or be willing to work on a BSN degree), and definitely had the clinical and leadership experience. I did not get the job. I decided to question the interviewer and specifically ask what qualifications she thought I lacked that prevented my being chosen. In order to not appear to be threatening, I softened my question with the comment that I'd like her feedback as I would like to work on those areas as a way of self-improvement, so that the next time such a position opened up, there would be no doubt about my qualifications. Oddly, she had no suggestions to offer other than to keep doing what I was doing. I don't know if the reason I didn't get the position was that being a Black man in a mid-level management position would be seen as threatening or if the interviewer had a personal agenda. As I recall, there were very few minorities in leadership positions at that time. The bottom line, as I saw it, was their loss was my gain. I accepted another position that I absolutely loved. As the outreach coordinator, I had the opportunity to educate students and other healthcare professionals regarding the care of burns, promote safety education, travel broadly, and conduct/promote safety research.

I think in my 44 years as a nurse, the most challenging job that I have held is my current job as the president of the American Nurses Association. Being elected as the first male president of an organization that had existed for 122 years with all female presidents (only two of whom were African American) certainly created a challenge and made me realize that everyone would be looking at me . . . waiting for me to make my first mistake. I realized that some of my colleagues would probably hope that I would fail, but I thought and felt that the majority of my colleagues would be very supportive and want me to succeed.

> *Being elected as the first male president of an organization that had existed for 122 years with all female presidents (only two of whom were African American) certainly created a challenge and made me realize that everyone would be looking at me . . . waiting for me to make my first mistake.*

There have been many, many challenges that I have had to face in this position, some very small and some very big. I think the most significant ones are:

- *Ensuring that nurses had the resources and education they needed to combat the pandemic:* This meant going before Congress, administrative agencies, and other healthcare agencies to plead our case.
- *Listening to nurses who are on the front line:* I established a group of 40 nurses across the country that work in a variety of settings that I speak with on a regular basis to gain insight about what is happening at the grassroots level. This helps me to be prepared when these issues become national issues.
- *The nursing workforce:* So many nurses are choosing to retire early, leave the profession, or become travelers. This has created quite a staffing issue for healthcare facilities and long-term care. I have written a letter to the secretary of health and human services calling for a declaration of a national crisis and to bring all players to the table so we can develop short- and long-term goals to address the nursing shortage. This cannot be solved overnight, but we need to start to work on this issue now if we are to save health and health care!
- *Social justice:* I strongly believe that as nurses we are advocates not only for our patients but also for our community. That being said, I also realize that what happens in our communities also affects the health and well-being of our community. That is why I feel it is so important for all nurses to become advocates within their community and have the sometimes tough dialogue to address social justice issues such as racism, access to care, and minority caregivers. This is the only way that we will be able to improve health and health care for all of us and not just a few!

I see the challenge ahead for the nursing profession in answering the question: What is nursing going to look like post-COVID? There have been some great strides made in some areas, but there has also been some regression. We definitely will not go back to what the profession looked like pre-COVID. The use of telehealth and telemedicine has made significant improvement in the management of chronic illnesses. It has given advanced practice nurses more autonomy and full practice authority. However, we also need to continue to advocate for the nurse at the bedside. I believe that we need to incorporate more innovation and technology that will allow nurses to work smarter, more efficiently and still be able to provide that much-needed hands-on care. Finally, I think it is imperative that nursing stop being treated as a commodity and be removed from the room-and-board charges for hospitalized patients and be allowed to bill for the care we provide. If our physician colleagues, pharmacists, physical therapists, and others can bill separately, why can't nurses? We must also start treating each other with respect and dignity. As the most trusted profession, we must do everything we can to maintain the public's trust and to make nursing the profession of choice for that young second or third grader who is thinking about what they would like to be when they grow up!

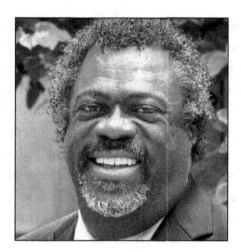

Ernest Grant, PhD, RN, FAAN

Dr. Ernest J. Grant is the 36th president of the American Nurses Association (ANA), the nation's largest nurse's organization representing the interests of the nation's 4.3 million registered nurses. He is the first man to be elected to the office of president of the ANA in its 125 years of existence.

An active participant in professional organizations, Grant is a past chair of the National Fire Protection Association board of directors and served as second vice president of the American Burn Association board of trustees. He also holds membership in Sigma Theta Tau and Chi Eta Phi. Grant served as president of the North Carolina Nurses Association from 2009 to 2011. In 2002, ANA honored Grant with the Honorary Nursing Practice Award for his contributions to the advancement of nursing practice through strength of character, commitment, and competence. In 2002, President George W. Bush presented Grant with a Nurse of the Year Award for his work treating burn victims from the World

Trade Center site. He was inducted as a fellow into the American Academy of Nursing in 2014. Grant holds a BSN degree from North Carolina Central University and MSN and PhD degrees from the University of North Carolina at Greensboro.

8

My Journey From Immigrant to Nurse Leader

Sun Jones, DNP, RN, FNP-BC

Why Did You Choose Nursing as a Career?

Nursing was not my first career choice, but it happened. Our family emigrated from South Korea to seek a better life. Many immigrant families come from oppression and poor conditions. South Korea was no different in the 1970s. After the Korean War, South Korea was still struggling to rise from the ashes of war. Our family, as well as others, suffered a great deal of financial hardship. My mother had to raise six children after my father died when I was only 11 years old. She had to find a way to come to the United States, a land of opportunity, for her children. She was a great seamstress; that helped us survive. My older sisters joined my mother in continuing their career in clothes-making and helped the family survive during those tough times.

The importance of education was strongly instilled by my mother. My mother did not receive much education during Japan's occupation of Korea. Because my grandfather was an educated man who resisted Japan's oppression, my grandfather and my uncle (my mother's brother) were killed, and their assets were seized. My mother was not allowed to attend school beyond her elementary education, but she instilled the importance of education in us and encouraged us to continue our education. Luckily, one of my older sisters and I came to the U.S. when we were in our teen years. I was able to attend 3 years of high school, which helped with my English. With help from my teachers and a counselor, I was able to continue my education at Arizona State University (ASU). I completed my first degree in microbiology but was not able to find a job to support myself. I went into business and continued with taking classes in business. I thought that I was better off with business, since many people who knew me said that I was very outgoing and would be perfect in the business field.

I like the term "things happen for reasons." It was not until my first child got ill and had many medical needs that I considered the option of a nursing career. I was working at a local bank 5 days a week and was trying to provide 24-hour care to my daughter. She was progressively getting worse with her neuromuscular issues. We tried many different specialists, but no one was able to find what was wrong with her. Due to her weakness, she was bedbound, was on oxygen, received tube feeding, and required suctioning to prevent aspiration. My sister, who was already an RN, suggested that I should become an RN so my schedule would be more flexible and I could become more knowledgeable in providing care to my daughter. I signed up at my alma mater and began taking nursing courses. Since I had a degree in microbiology, I was able to start the program right away. Looking back, I vaguely remember the process, but I remember that it was rather easy. Having a science degree from

> I chose nursing as my career to take care of my ill child, but it changed my entire life.

the same institution definitely made things much easier. I particularly remember having a coordinator who helped guide me through the entire admission process and helped me gather all necessary documents.

While attending school, I took a job as a nurse extern at the Phoenix Children's Hospital so I could learn what to expect when I became a nurse. I really enjoyed learning, and it was the beginning of my nursing career.

The mastery of language skills to work in the medical field is something that all immigrants are challenged to acquire.

After graduating from nursing school, I found out there are so many opportunities in many different fields for nurses. I explored other options while preparing to start an NP program. I chose nursing as my career to take care of my ill child, but it changed my entire life.

Progression and Challenges in the Program

The progression schedule was laid out, and we had to follow it. I am a systems-thinking person and have organization skills that helped me through the BSN and MSN programs. For me, the challenges were, and still are, the language skills. I was proud to say that I had great math skills which helped with science and technology. When applying those skills, I found them very easy to learn and adapt to. Applying my limited language skill was another level of challenge and learning. The mastery of language skills to work in the medical field is something that all immigrants are challenged to acquire.

Share About Your First Job and Your Career Progression

Challenges

After graduation, we were all told that hospitals did not have much need for new graduates. Even the hospital where I was working as an extern did not have positions available for new graduates. There was no shortage of nurses. However, I was very lucky to be offered a job at one of the biggest trauma centers in the valley. I started working on the medical–surgical floor, as recommended by my faculty and preceptors. I was very task oriented and had great skills in multitasking. This was a great asset in working at a very busy hospital. Working on a medical–surgical floor helped me learn about disease processes and treatments. However, much of the caring that I was supposed do was replaced with tasks such as bathing, passing out medications, and hanging IV medications, etc. The work was very physically demanding and mentally exhausting. I had moments of satisfaction of being a nurse, but it was no different than working at a factory trying to meet my quota for that one day.

Opportunities

Having a nursing degree provided me with many opportunities. I realized that I could become and do whatever I wish to do with my nursing degree. Before I graduated from the BSN program, one of the assistant deans pulled me aside and asked if I would come back to the school for the NP degree. I smiled and said, "Okay" but I did not take her seriously. One night after a 12-hour shift of running like a hamster in a wheel, I decided to place a call to the school. I obtained an introduction to the FNP (family nurse practitioner) program and information about what was required. I began looking at other roles as a nurse within the institution where I was working so my schedule could accommodate my personal life and school. During this exploration, I found many different areas where I could work with my BSN. I realized that there is a lot more than floor nursing.

Milestones

I took on a role of case manager. The work schedule was more conducive to attending the night classes the school offered: there was no high-speed internet and Google did not exist. This was another learning point. As a case manager, I worked with physicians and rounded with them. I learned about the disease process and how they decided to care for the patients. I learned about utilization review, insurance, and community resources, which helped me a great deal during my career as a nurse practitioner.

After becoming an FNP, I continued to precept students so I could remain current in what was going on in academia. I was hesitant to continue with my degree to become a doctor of nursing practice (DNP), but I chose to start and completed this work in 2010. I have not had any regrets after I received the DNP degree.

After receiving a DNP degree, I was contacted by a local university to teach a course. Since then, other nursing opportunities have opened up for me. Moving from a faculty member to an administrator was another path that was presented to me. I saw more opportunities at a higher level as a program and curriculum evaluator.

Current Role

Currently, I serve as a program and curriculum evaluator. However, I was the program chair for the MSN/FNP program.

Challenges

Being in the nursing program did not prepare me to become a leader. A leader must have certain qualities but needs to grow into a position through learning leadership skills. As a first-generation immigrant, my biggest challenge was the language. For some people, learning language may come very easily. The transition from being a lay language speaker to writing, speaking, and presenting at a much higher level of professionalism was the biggest challenge for me. I did not have a mentor to help me grow as a leader in the beginning. I remember being identified to become a leader when I was working for a local bank prior to working as a nurse, purely due to my ethnicity. During my early career as a nurse, I was not presented with any nursing leadership opportunities, nor did I have any confidence to be a leader. Through my education, I learned about leadership. I was always shy and lacked confidence due to my language skill. It resulted in my doing more tasks to support the leaders. I was praised on how well I completed my work. This built my confidence in working on tasks, but I still did not realize that there were so many skills that I had to learn to be a leader.

> *Equity means giving the same opportunities to all, not just based on race, gender, or any other characteristics.*

Opportunities

I am grateful for the opportunity to live in this country and all the opportunities that have been laid out in front of me. Some I sought out, but some were presented in front of me during my career. I was given opportunities because of being Asian, but those did not last long. I felt like they had to include me to meet their numbers and government mandate. I rejected those opportunities, and my resentment grew since I felt like I was invited to be one of the statistics. However, when the opportunities were presented with recognition of my work experience as an NP and my educational background, I felt the sense of belonging and appreciation.

Your Recommendations for Equity in the Future

Equity means giving the same opportunities to all, not just based on race, gender, or any other characteristics. Inclusion of many minorities must start early, not while in their professional roles. Schools and educators must present the leadership roles to all students and provide them with skills. Many immigrant children may not be able to see the vision of becoming a leader or have the opportunity to dream of leadership roles; they may be struggling to survive as I did.

If we treat each other as people, not by their gender, color or ethnicity, we can truly say we are all equal.

As educators, we should look at the potential in each person and develop their leadership skills. It is not so much for giving them opportunities to be a leader, but allowing them to start developing their leadership skills through classwork.

To increase inclusion and diversity, leaders must identify the needs of the minority groups. Their needs and path to becoming a leader will be different than the traditional pathway.

If we treat each other as people, not by their gender, color or ethnicity, we can truly say we are all equal.

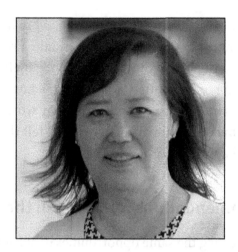

Sun Jones, DNP, RN, FNP-BC

Sun Jones is a doctor of nursing practice (DNP)-prepared and board-certified family nurse practitioner (FNP). She earned her DNP in 2010 and MSN/FNP in 2001 from Arizona State University. She currently works as a systematic plan of evaluation and curriculum evaluator and an associate faculty member and practices as a family nurse practitioner. As an immigrant, she focused on providing primary care to Koreans who have been challenged with multiple barriers. Sun has mentored many nurses to follow her beliefs in the importance of educating nurses to improve the overall health of the general population. She also actively leads and volunteers in many community organizations. With grants and fundings she has received, she has been helping not only the Korean community but also the Arizona Asian Pacific Islander communities by providing health screenings and supporting vaccination efforts.

9

Nursing Across Three Countries and Two Continents

Aniko Kukla, DNP, RN, CPNP

Colleagues I look up to and admire have wonderful stories to tell. From their early childhood, they wanted to be a nurse because there was someone or a situation that inspired them. I was always envious of their inspiration, and though I lacked an early role model, I undertook a decade-long journey that ended with a DNP. I will continue to cherish for the rest of my career the insight and understanding I gain in this wonderful career that is never-ending.

I grew up in what was formerly called Yugoslavia in the 1970s. Subotica, my hometown, was a midsize industrial suburb in northern Serbia south of the Hungarian border. Subotica was a multicultural city with a mixture of various ethnicities, nationalities, and religions. In my early childhood, communism was gasping for its last breath, but the economy was still somewhat strong. People were living stable lives, the factories were open, and families could rely on a steady income. We were able to attend schools as ethnic minorities in our mother tongue (Hungarian), though from early childhood we had to learn the official language of the country (Serbian) and an additional foreign language apart from Hungarian (usually German or English). During my early childhood, I remember vacationing at the Adriatic Sea and spending the days running around my grandparents' farm watching my grandma prep her produce to sell at the local farmers market. I remember watching her run after me with a ladder when I would get stuck in the fruit trees. I was not brave enough to jump off, but she always made me feel like I was the most important thing at the moment, and her duty was to save me.

My grandmother would get up at 5 a.m. and load her produce on her bike, although she never learned to ride it. She would push the bike for an hour to get to her stall at the market by 6 a.m. Both of my parents were factory workers. Dad stopped going to school in sixth grade, and my mother (although she wanted to study to become a kindergarten teacher) had to attend trade school to become a worker in the sock factory, as her family could not afford to send her to school. I never realized that we were from a less than affluent family, as my mother always made it clear that there were many families that were much poorer than we were. Indeed, there were many kids I knew who came to school hungry. In second grade, my parents got divorced and the economy tanked. I remember that buying food and necessities was a struggle but also that no one in my family complained. My mother kept working in the factory, but due to Yugoslavia's hyperinflation, by the time she cashed her check the money was worth half of what it was worth earlier that same day. Many times, there were long lines at the bank, and the bank would often run out of money. As a result, my mother was often only able to pay the monthly mortgage and maybe would have enough left over to buy a loaf of bread. It seems like we were always standing in line for something (be it detergent, coffee, sugar, etc.). Inflation was out of control, and new bills were printed by the treasury monthly. We had millions, even billions of currency (Yugoslavian dinars) lying around the house that were not worth a penny. We used to joke that we were the world's poorest billionaires. Despite this, I was never hungry, cold, or suffered from lack of any basic needs. I think it was my family's attitude that helped us to persevere: I was always told the glass is half full, not half empty.

By the end of the 1980s, nationalism was on the rise, and we would hear about the daily ethnic fights in the other parts of the country (now known as Croatia, Bosnia and Herzegovina, and Kosovo). Yet somehow, our city was still under a bubble of disbelief that a tragic civil war was imminent. I suppose everyone was in collective denial, as this was our most successful survival tactic. Inevitably, though, reality displaces denial, and strong people resort to stoic determination as their only means to survive.

Inevitably, though, reality displaces denial, and strong people resort to stoic determination as their only means to survive.

As long as I can remember, my mother always hustled a side gig in addition to her full-time job, and she never complained about doing so. She told me that my only job was "to study and do well in life." One day in sixth grade, my advisory teacher decided to visit all the families in his class at their homes. When he visited my house, I remember him saying to my mother that he did not understand how one of his best students could live in a house that was the size of a shoebox and with no running water. To which my mother replied, "The last I checked, knowledge did not drip through the faucet but was coming from books." I was amused and mortified at the same time as I saw my teacher running out the door, shaking his head in disbelief.

In Yugoslavia, the education system was set up to have students choose between a specialized vocational high school or a general high school focused on college prep by the end of eighth grade. The strongest schools in the city were the nursing high school and the "gymnasium," the college prep school. I had no idea at age 14 what I wanted to be; I just knew I wanted to help people. Whenever I heard my family talk about education, they would say something to the extent of "Education is a way out of poverty, and the ticket out of the country."

I grew up watching *L.A. Law*, a TV series from the 1980s that had a healthy dose of drama and comedy. It featured lawyers dealing with socially viable topics and portrayed the law as a socially responsible profession. The show's characters dealt with hot topics like gay rights, AIDS, abortion, and racism. The show explored the ambiguity of these topics in depth (or at least with as much depth as a teenager in a somewhat sheltered life could understand). Later, I was not surprised to learn that this show is believed to have led to an increase in law school applications. I still believe this show's worldwide impact is understated.

L.A. Law convinced me that serving humanity was my calling. I wanted to vigorously pursue law until multiple family members warned me that a law degree is country specific. They correctly advised me that if I moved to another country I would be doing dishes, as a Serbian law degree would not be worth much outside of Yugoslavia. Still, I wanted to serve humanity, and so I explored my other option, nursing, and went to Subotica's vocational nursing school at age 14. My family seemed more excited about my prospects with a nursing degree as they thought it would be something that I could always fall back on and it would allow me to find gainful employment outside of Yugoslavia. I remember getting my first uniform and hilarious open-toe, white, lace-up shoes (no idea what the workers' protection union was thinking at the time), heading out to the wards for clinicals, and feeling such pride that I was joining a noble profession that would allow me to help humanity in the same way I watched the lawyers on *L.A. Law* help and sacrifice for the greater good.

I remember agonizing for days upon graduation from high school about a choice that would change my life forever: Was I to attend the medical university free (accepted with a full scholarship) in Yugoslavia or leave the country to go to Hungary on a scholarship, but with it be required to attend preparatory school and risk not getting into medical school? My family was worried that the ethnic clashes would turn into a civil war, and as medical students we would be pulled into taking care of the wounded. They strongly advised me to leave the country. Additionally, I felt that this war was something I did not believe in. Civil war is ugly; neighbors started hating each other just because they were from different ethnic backgrounds. I could not acquiesce to the logic of hate that was prevailing.

Thus, I made the very difficult decision to leave my family and my place at the medical university and move to Hungary. It quickly became evident that my primary and secondary education was subpar, leaving many holes in the foundation of my knowledge. For the first time in my life, school was hard, and I was struggling to keep up. I had 10 months to learn chemistry, physics, and biology at the superior Hungarian acumen (of course the Hungarians had 4 years to develop their acuity). Although my scholarship paid for the dorm and food and gave us a bit of a stipend, it was still only enough for the necessities. However, I felt very lucky. At home, the war preparations were indeed progressing, my male family members were called to serve in the army reserves, and most of the factories closed down. Life was miserable, and I somehow escaped all this. While others were fighting, I was able to take long walks around Budapest and sit on the banks of the Danube and dream about the future.

My plan to get into the medical university did not work out, as I missed passing the entrance exam by one point. I did successfully gain entrance to the Hungarian nursing program, however. The BSN program that my application defaulted to was in the western part of Hungary in the city called Zalaegerszeg. I had never heard of this city, and I had to buy a map to find out where it was. Still, I was devastated. I was going back to a nursing school, but in my mind, I was already a nurse. I wanted to become a physician, and I looked at the nursing program as a default placeholder until I could get into the medical university. I felt I was better than this and nursing was just a waste of time.

To make matters worse, Zalaegerszeg ended up being a city far away from my hometown, a day's travel including two trains and a bus. Getting to and from the college required money and time, two things that I was in short supply of. Furthermore, as a newcomer to this city and college, I acquired all kinds of new labels: "foreigner," "Yugoslav," and "out-of-city kid." I was never invited into the local college kids' homes. The other "out-of-town" kids from other cities disappeared on the weekends. Many times, I was roaming the halls of the dorm by myself and wondering what the future would bring. Things back home were going from bad to worse. The economy in Yugoslavia was in shambles, and my mother decided to follow me to Hungary. She moved into a workers' hostel after getting a job in one of the local factories in a nearby town. Again, we were struggling financially, but considered ourselves very lucky that

> *As a newcomer to this city and college, I acquired all kinds of new labels: "foreigner," "Yugoslav," and "out-of-city kid."*

we were able to get out of the country and did not have to endure the daily stresses of the horrible economy that many of our relatives and family members had to. We were able to meet up on the weekends and support each other emotionally. We watched old movies and cooked some food for the week ahead.

To occupy myself on days off and when college was not in session, I got a couple of jobs: I was a dishwasher, a cleaning lady, and then was promoted to a security guard at the nursing school. It required me to do a walk-through, lock the doors at 10:00 p.m., watch some TV, sleep (a perk of this job was that the night shift was allowed to go to sleep—they even gave us pillows and blankets), and get up at 6:00 a.m. to open the door for the workers and professors. I was so lucky; I had a job that afforded me the time to figure out what I wanted to do with my life. During this time, I became friends with the other security guards, the cleaning crew, and the librarian, all who have unknowingly helped me figure things out. They shared with me the immense sense of pride regarding their stake in "raising the next generation of nurses," and I then realized how foolish I was to think that being a nurse was somewhat beneath me.

Little did I know when I signed up to study at this remote location that I was signing up for one of the first BSN programs in Hungary where the curriculum was to be aligned with the 4-year BSN curriculum at Case Western Reserve University in Cleveland, Ohio. During my freshman year, an older couple visited the nursing college from the United States. We had to appear at their reception and wear our best clothing. The program directors told us that these people were the benefactors of the program. One of them was a professor of nursing studies and had a doctorate in nursing, something that we had never heard of before. This professor's mission was to help elevate nursing to a professional level in Hungary.

She told us that there would be opportunities for us to visit where she worked and see how nursing is practiced. I remember sitting in the farthest corner of the auditorium and whispering into my friend's ear jokingly, "Watch me; one day I will do that!"

For 2 years in a row, I fought to get into the medical university in Hungary, not giving up my original dream of becoming a physician. The entrance exam consisted of both written and oral exams in two subjects, physics and biology. The day of the oral exam at the medical university was one of the most exhausting, frightening, and humiliating experiences in my life. While it taught me a big lesson in equity, it also propelled me further toward my goal than I could have ever imagined. During the oral exam, one had to pick an envelope from the table that contained a topic from biology and physics and present to the board of 5 college professors what they knew about it, after which the professors could ask any question they liked. My exam started with my red Yugoslavian passport being passed around and a professor exclaiming, "Aha, another foreigner from Yugoslavia trying to get in." The rest is history.

> *I remember sitting in the farthest corner of the auditorium and whispering into my friend's ear jokingly, "Watch me; one day I will do that!"*

I did not do well, not because they tried to humiliate me by pointing out that I was a foreigner trying to pick up a free ride, not because they asked why I would switch from nursing to medicine, and not because they wondered why nursing was not good enough for me. I did not do well because I had sold myself short. I believed that I was less than the native-born Hungarians were, and I was ashamed of my background. I also believed I was doomed to fail because my education was inferior. I remember I could not recite the planets in order (although I did describe in detail how enzymes worked, as biology came naturally to me). Years later, I was chuckling to myself when Pluto was demoted after I was promoted at work. After failing to get into medical school again, I realized I had two choices: continue with nursing school or try again to transfer and go to medical school. It was here that I decided I would be the best nurse I could possibly become.

I was finally ready to apply myself and focus on nursing. I studied hard and immersed myself in foundational subjects like psychology in order to get to know myself. I studied and shared notes and insights with other students. I remember standing at the photocopier for hours copying from medical textbooks because we did not have our own textbooks, as we were the first 4-year nursing school with an updated curriculum. When the call to apply for a scholarship to visit Case Western University College of Nursing came, I jumped on the opportunity. One of the requirements was that we pass a national certification exam in English language. I studied day

> *It was here that I decided I would be the best nurse I could possibly become.*

and night and traveled for hours by bus to get to the exam center to take the test. One of the best days of my life was when I found out I passed the exam and received the scholarship. As I was celebrating with friends who had also passed, it dawned on me that I was still not one of them; I had a red passport from my new postwar country Serbia, which was relegated to the U.S. visa watchlist for the atrocities they committed during the war. For days, I was thinking about how I could make my passport less red so it blended in with the blue Hungarian passports.

I organized the trip to the embassy with all of the students in my cohort who were also accepted for this trip, hoping that this would provide me with some kind of advantage. The entire time I was at the embassy, I was highly anxious, hoping that maybe my passport would be overlooked and ignored because it was among their more desirable passports. Maybe, just maybe, they would look at me as a Hungarian from Hungary and not a Yugoslavian turned into a Serbian. In the end, all the blue passport Hungarian students received 10-year visas. I, on the other hand, was grilled repeatedly. They continually asked what I was planning to do in Cleveland and if I was coming back to Hungary. After more than an hour, I was finally granted a travel visa that was valid for one year. I was frustrated but still claimed victory: I got a visa.

In Cleveland, a new world opened to me as soon as I arrived. I saw what a noble profession nursing was outside of Hungary. The nursing textbooks and journals in the medical library, how nurses were empowered to use critical thinking, and the integral part they have played in their patients' lives all solidified my resolve that I was in a noble profession and this was the perfect profession for me. The 3 weeks I spent in Cleveland, Ohio, as a visiting student changed my life. I had come to establish a new dream: I would come back to the United States and one day receive a doctorate in nursing.

When I got back to Hungary, there was a lot to do. We had to write a thesis, complete a research study, and do a 6-month internship at the local hospital. One time during the night shift, I was told that I had to "hold down the fort" with the nursing assistant until the morning. There we were, just the two of us attending to 26 patients. We were handed a long list of tasks: pass medications out, feed and change the patients, tuck them in, and care for patients who needed extra attention. Under no circumstance were we to wake up the doctor before 5:00 a.m., unless a patient was dying, and even then, I was warned that we "better have coffee in your hand when the doctor arrives" (they were dead serious about this). I was told more staff would be arriving at 6:00 a.m. for the morning baths. I remember saying a prayer in my head over and over, hoping that all the patients would be okay and survive until the morning. I am still not sure who was more scared, me or my assistant. We made it through the night without having to wake up the physician. That night only strengthened my resolution: Despite not being fluent in English, not knowing how I would get into the nursing school, and not knowing how I was going to pay for the studies, I was going back to Cleveland.

Throughout my journey, I encountered many angels but none more significant to my success than the professor who sponsored the trip we took to Cleveland, Ohio. She eventually became my mentor, and with the support of the Hungarian community, I was able to start the MSN program at the University of Akron.

At first, it was hard. It took me an hour to read one page of an article with a dictionary and days to write a one- or two-page assignment. I had to think of what the professor might ask about the topic when I was studying for class because by the time I translated the question in my head and formulated the answer, the class had already moved on to the next topic of discussion. Over time, I came to realize that while everything was possible, I needed to develop the strength and stamina to stick with the process. This is why I love this country and nursing. There are many avenues one can take and still succeed; all you need is determination.

Sometime at the end of my first year in the MSN program, the administration decided that a requirement to continue with the program was a one-year nursing internship in a hospital setting. I was able to find a pediatric nursing job at the prestigious Cleveland

Clinic with the help of the Hungarian community, but my paperwork was a mess. Obtaining an off-campus internship required coordination from the nursing school, the university's international office, and the hospital's human resources department.

I think this was my first experience with attempting to coordinate a project between siloed, bureaucratic systems that are not set up to effectively communicate with each other. A week before my visa was to expire, I called the international office at my school. I was overwhelmed with anxiety and was crying, and I did not know how to solve the issue. Different people were sending me around in circles, and I was told I would be "shipped back home" if my paperwork was not in order (this is exactly what one administrator of the school told me). A young administrator helped me by getting all involved parties together so that they could agree on what exactly needed to be done. Years later, this man would become my loving husband. He loves to tell the story of how he saved my life. Little did he know at the time that he was not just doing his job. His compassion for a stranger indeed saved my life. He also did not know that I would, in turn, greatly influence the course of his life.

At the Cleveland Clinic, the preceptors and nurses were, for the most part, welcoming. They taught me not just about how to be a nurse but also socialized me to the healthcare culture. I learned a lot from the seasoned nurses on the night shift. They were great role models and taught me how to approach physicians, how to talk to patients and families, and most importantly how to be a strong advocate for patients. One of my fondest memories involves one seasoned nurse who was not especially friendly, who was difficult to connect with, and who rarely showed her human side. I watched her care for a teenage boy who suffered from uncontrollable seizures. I witnessed her administer his medication and then immediately drop to her knees hugging and holding him, telling him everything would be okay and that she was with him so he should not worry because she wouldn't let anything bad happen to him. Though he was unable to move, this boy had tears rolling down his cheeks. This seasoned nurse demonstrated to me that even behind the hardest shell, a good nurse has a soft heart that cares about their patients. This is why we became nurses: to be there and help people when they need us the most. This was another moment of affirmation for me: I was in the right profession. I could make a difference by being there for people who needed me.

Even behind the hardest shell, a good nurse has a soft heart that cares about their patients.

I continued to be employed as a nurse in Cleveland for more than 15 years. I have been a staff nurse in the pediatric, vascular, and bariatric nursing units. I have also worked as an educator and quality/Magnet® manager at both large hospitals and smaller community hospitals. I have learned a lot about humility, cultural norms, and expectations. My career was advancing at a great clip. Suddenly I suffered a major setback (or at least I thought it was at the time). In 2012, the economy suffered a great shock and hospitals started cutting back on spending. Naturally, nursing departments had to cut as well. Through several coincidences and circumstances, I found myself unemployed and unable to secure a job, as all hiring seemed to be frozen indefinitely. I ended up collecting unemployment and became depressed. I did not know how to deal with all the feelings that began to surface. I blamed and beat myself up over my situation. There were many things I did not understand that I do now: specifically, how organizations work and how upper-level decisions are made.

It was then that I met another angel on my road to success. One nurse leader took me under her wing. She picked me up, dusted me off, and talked me into accepting a low-paying clinical instructor position, which I reluctantly accepted. I was frustrated as I had to deduct my small stipend from my unemployment check. I was also questioning the logic of accepting this part-time position, as I thought I should be trying to find a full-time job. What I did not understand was that this part-time clinical instructor position would force me to get out of bed, put my uniform on, and get to work teaching nursing students. Being employed again helped me to regain my sense of purpose and improve my outlook on life. This position was integral to the wisdom this nurse leader was trying to convey: Setbacks are a normal part of life, and by losing a job (which I realized was consuming me), I found a new outlook. I learned to take care of myself physically and mentally, and in the end, I got an opportunity to finish my doctoral studies.

> *Setbacks are a normal part of life, and by losing a job (which I realized was consuming me), I found a new outlook.*

I worked my way up to clinical instructor supervisor in one of the area's associate degree programs and found myself working with some of the best nurses in the area. Many of them were also employed in area hospitals and were working as clinical instructors as a way of giving back to the nursing profession. I soon realized what a gift it was to have the chance to influence others. Nursing, yet again, provided me with an opportunity I may not otherwise have been able to have: the opportunity to work with and influence students from all backgrounds. Some were young, fresh out of high school, concerned with what they would be doing after school, and what party they would attend. Others were single moms or dads, sometimes working full time elsewhere or working odd jobs so they would be able to afford nursing school and pay for the necessities of their families. Some were from the poor areas of Cleveland where they had feared for their kids' safety on the street daily; some came from affluent lives but suddenly had to learn how to take care of themselves. At the bedside and in our uniforms, we all became the same: a nurse who was there to help the patient. We soon managed to understand each other. These ADN students proved to be more highly motivated and harder working than many master's- or doctoral-level students I encountered. They inspired me to take my career to the next level.

Inspired by the students I met, I soon signed up to study quality and safety at the Veterans Administration Hospital in the VA Quality Scholarship Program. This led me to set sail into uncharted waters and embark on a career in hospital administration in Salinas, California, where I am leading the quality processes at the Salinas Valley Memorial Hospital. This is a hospital where I can learn and grow every day and where I am supported to be my best every day. This is a hospital where I can support my team of employees in the same way my career mentors have supported me.

In my current role as a leader in quality, I have the opportunity again of working with some of the most highly motivated and engaged bedside nurses and leaders I have ever had the privilege to encounter. It is inspiring to me that I can empower them to take charge of their own practice by participating in continuous improvement. We all have two roles in our profession; one is to do our jobs and the other is to do better for our patients.

There is a growing need to provide more equitable health care, and this starts by providing equitable nursing education. Equitable nursing education will only be possible if we have enough qualified faculty ready to teach these concepts. I hope that many of my colleagues will step up and start teaching, either in nursing schools or by being preceptors at the bedside to raise the future generation of nurses. This would not only benefit the students and patients but also nurses themselves. So many great nurses are currently experiencing burnout syndrome and considering leaving the profession forever. Teaching could be a way to reinvigorate themselves so they can inspire others.

> *Equitable nursing education will only be possible if we have enough qualified faculty ready to teach these concepts.*

In many ways my studies across three countries and two continents was like time traveling. I started with a healthcare structure in Eastern Europe that resembled the current U.S. system 30 to 40 years ago. By moving through different countries and education systems, I was exposed to different practices and philosophies, all of which have their own set of challenges but all of which uniquely influenced me. What I learned from the nurses in Yugoslavia and Hungary is that it is possible to practice health care and to be a great nurse with less than state-of-the-art equipment. What I have come to understand from working with colleagues in the United States is that at the bedside we are all equal and that in an emergency, no one is looking at race, ethnicity,

> *My studies across three countries and two continents was like time traveling.*

or country of origin. Once we are graduated and at the bedside, we are all colleagues, and in a moment of crisis there is only one thing that matters, and that is that the patient survives and does well.

In summary, I hope I have portrayed the following ideas:

- Whether you choose to believe you will fail or you choose to believe you will succeed, you are right.
- As long as there are problems, solutions can be found.
- Teach children from an early age how not to be victims.
- Positive role models are important.
- When you feel you are poor or less than others, know that there are people whose situation is worse than yours.
- Students who have had to surmount the biggest hurdles often become the strongest nurses.
- Demonstrate to children and demoralized adults the importance of refocusing their visions. A strong goal will guide you like a lighthouse on a dark sea.
- If a girl with a heavy accent who was reading articles with a dictionary and took hours to read a page of an article can accomplish her lofty goals, then you can too!

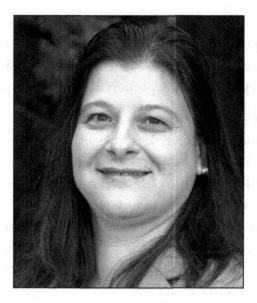

Aniko Kukla, DNP, RN, CPNP

Aniko Kukla, DNP, RN, CPNP, is a quality and safety professional, institutional negotiator, medical writer, and improvement coach, but most importantly, a nurse. Currently she heads Quality and Safety at Salinas Valley Memorial Hospital, where she oversees quality reporting and performance improvement. Passionate about lifelong learning, Dr. Kukla is a strong advocate for advanced studies in nursing. She is a graduate of Case Western Reserve University Frances Payne Bolton School of Nursing, where she received her doctor of nursing practice in 2013. In addition, she graduated from The University of Akron master of science program as a pediatric nurse practitioner. She began her education in Pecs, Hungary, where she received a bachelor of science degree in nursing. Dr. Kukla is a former Magnet Program manager and nurse educator who has learned that there is no stronger inspiration than supporting and empowering bedside nurses. It is here that she sees the greatest opportunity to create innovations and sustainable improvements. She is currently a cochair for the International Subcommittee at the Quality and Safety Nursing Education Institute. Dr. Kukla is also a highly regarded subject matter expert for many nursing education textbooks and modules. In her free time, she can be found having a good debate with her two teenagers and husband or reading a good book on the beach in Monterey, CA.

10

Learn to Become the Learner

John Lowe, PhD, RN, FAAN

Overcoming Barriers and Breaking Stereotypes

My story begins in the Southeast in a small Native American community consisting of a few families. My father, who was Cherokee and Creek, never attended school himself but inspired me and my siblings to pursue education. My mother, who was of Lenape tribal ancestry, passed away when I was young. She attended a small tribal school from grades one to seven.

I initially had to overcome barriers of racial discrimination to become a nurse—a career I chose in high school after relatives, some of whom were nurses themselves, suggested it. Because of the influence of my grandmother and other relatives, I became interested in helping people, and I was described by relatives to be caring of others and their needs, including the animals and plants that lived among us. My high school had a licensed practical nurse (LPN) program that I enrolled in during my junior year. I did this upon the advice of a school counselor, who leaned across her desk one day and said, "To become a registered nurse (RN) means going to college; people where you are from [Native Americans] don't go to college." The counselor suggested the LPN program or some other "service career" would be the appropriate options for me to pursue. She also suggested that I begin by working as an orderly (a male nursing assistant). So, I said to myself, "I guess that's what I have to do." While studying in the LPN program as a junior and senior high school student, I worked as an orderly in the local hospital and nursing home on weekends and school breaks/vacations. This provided me the funds I needed to purchase the extra materials needed for the LPN program. It also provided me with an expanded experience to practice the skills I was learning in the LPN program. Upon graduating high school, I passed the licensure exam to become an LPN, and I worked at the local hospital for 3 years. With the encouragement of coworkers, I searched for small colleges with BSN programs located within a few hours from home. I applied and was accepted to a small, private, religious-affiliated college in Virginia. Being a first-generation college student within my family, I had to navigate this endeavor without the foresight or knowledge of those around me. As a result of my previous experience with being stereotyped in high school and the fear of being denied the opportunity to pursue a college degree, I kept my identity as a Native American very quiet. I felt that in order to survive this educational pursuit, my identity as a Native American had to become "invisible." This strategy seemed to work, as I was able to gain the confidence needed to be successful academically. I explored leadership opportunities, such as being elected as president of the Student Nurses Association. These experiences reaffirmed that being invisible had worked and contributed to my success in earning the BSN. However, deep within my spirit, I knew I had sacrificed disclosing and living openly as who I was as a Native American.

Taking Advantage of Opportunities

One of my first experiences providing health care came immediately after earning the BSN, when, as part of a Health Care

Missions program, I worked in Tanzania East Africa in mission hospitals assisting in surgery and with a mobile health clinic that offered maternal and child health care. I actually felt somewhat at home within the tribal settings reminiscent of my own childhood tribal culture environment. This broadened my perspective of the world and the possible opportunities as an RN. After returning from Tanzania, I accepted my first job as a staff nurse, working in the orthopedic unit at a local hospital in southeast Virginia. As a staff nurse, I also looked for various opportunities to become involved at different levels. I volunteered to be a preceptor for nursing students and new employees at the hospital along with volunteering to speak at local high schools to share about the kind of opportunities that a career in nursing could provide for men, especially minority men. Within a couple of years, I relocated to Oklahoma, desiring to be among extended family and live again within a Native American community. I applied and was accepted into the master's in nursing (MSN) program at a local university. While pursuing the MSN, I also worked at the university hospital—first as a medical/surgical staff nurse, then in an administrative position. Knowing the issues related to substance use among Native Americans, I eventually moved to a position in the hospital's substance abuse unit, working with adolescents who were struggling with alcohol and drug use and addiction—an experience that would ultimately give direction for my future research career. After receiving the MSN degree, I began teaching at the university. During the next few years, I began focusing on providing health care to diverse and underserved populations. I worked with international students at the university as an advisor, served as a community health instructor for senior nursing students who were assigned to community health experiences within local Native American tribes, and traveled to China, Jamaica, and Costa Rica, where I provided primary care and taught health promotion and disease prevention. I eventually moved to Florida to pursue a PhD in nursing at a university that had a transcultural nursing research focus. At the same time, I continued to work at various psychiatric/mental health facilities, gaining more experience in the area of treatment and therapies for substance use issues among various diverse populations. It became apparent to me that culturally appropriate interventions were not available for members of diverse populations who were seeking treatment. Especially lacking were treatments appropriate for those who were Native American. Leadership opportunities and possibilities to represent Native American and Indigenous people have come in many forms and venues. For example, having been a predoctoral fellow within the Minority Fellowship Program (MFP) at the American Nurses Association (ANA) and supported by the Substance Abuse Mental Health Services Administration, I later became a member and chair of the National Advisory Committee to the MFP.

> *Culturally appropriate interventions were not available for members of diverse populations who were seeking treatment. Especially lacking were treatments appropriate for those who were Native American.*

Several other opportunities have emerged, including serving as a member of the National Advisory Council to the National Institutes of Nursing Research at the National Institutes of Health. I have learned that it is very important to be "at the table" to have a voice to advocate for Native American/Indigenous people, as most "tables" do not have Native American nursing representation.

Research with a Purpose

During my PhD studies, I began to give more thought to investigating why my father had managed to avoid substance use and other serious health problems common to Native Americans. I gained more insight into my father's ability to integrate his Native American culture and traditions into his daily life. Unlike many other Native Americans growing up in the early 20th century, my father did not attend one of the infamous

> *It is very important to be "at the table" to have a voice to advocate for Native American/Indigenous people, as most "tables" do not have Native American nursing representation.*

boarding schools that were designed to assimilate Native American people into the White majority culture by separating them from their families and communities. My father's eldest sister had attended a boarding school and experienced the abuse and trauma perpetrated against most Native American children who attended boarding schools. As a result, my father and his other siblings avoided being sent to the boarding schools, which resulted in no formal education. The boarding schools for Native American children were first established in 1878, when Captain Richard H. Pratt opened the Carlisle Indian School at an abandoned military post in Pennsylvania (Kliewer et al., n.d.). Pratt's goal was to assimilate Native American children into the colonized Western culture by forcing them to abandon their Native culture—a concept he called "killing the Indian, not the man [person]." The boarding schools were deliberately located far away from tribal communities, and

Native children and their families were discouraged from visiting one another. The students were forbidden to speak their language or practice their spirituality, and they were told that the Native way of life was savage and inferior. Students often were required to wear military uniforms and were severely beaten for violating rules.

Those who returned to their Native American communities after leaving boarding school often found they had a hard time fitting in and exhibited behaviors that result from having experienced trauma. They had been stripped of their Native culture and identity by their experience in the boarding schools. My father's escape from the boarding school experience contributed to him having the opportunity to live in an environment where he learned tribal traditions, values, and beliefs.

The Cherokee Self-Reliance theoretical framework and model emerged from this research. Since then, this framework and model has expanded to other tribes and Indigenous people globally and has emerged to become the Native-Reliance theoretical framework and model.

As I pursued the PhD degree, it became clear to me that my father was able to stay physically and mentally healthy because he had not been dispossessed of his culture and heritage. He knew who he was, which gave him a sense of balance and harmony. So, it stood to reason that Native American young people suffering from substance use problems might be helped by incorporating Native American cultural traditions into their lives. My doctoral dissertation focused on using an ethnographic research method to describe the cultural mainstay of Cherokees, which investigated the connection between traditional Cherokee values and the health of Cherokee people. The Cherokee Self-Reliance theoretical framework and model emerged from this research (Lowe, 2002). Since then, this framework and model has expanded to other tribes and Indigenous people globally and has emerged to become the Native-Reliance theoretical framework and model (Lowe et al., 2019).

After completing the PhD degree, I obtained a faculty position that involved teaching full time. Conducting research was an added activity that most faculty chose not to invest time doing. Desiring to obtain more knowledge and expertise regarding quantitative methods, intervention development, and using randomized control trial designs, I applied and was accepted for a postdoctoral fellowship position with a clinical psychologist mentor who had expertise in substance use intervention research. The postdoctoral fellowship provided funding to support my salary and research activities. However, the dean of the nursing school where I was faculty insisted that I continue teaching a full load of courses. I complied with her demand and continued teaching all of the courses I was assigned, along with focusing on developing a substance use intervention, the Talking Circle, that incorporated the cultural concepts from my dissertation (Lowe et al., 2016). The intervention was implemented and tested among a sample of Cherokee youth. Findings revealed the intervention was useful for reducing substance interest and use along with decreasing stress, anxiety, and depression. Additionally, cultural identity and school performance improved among the participants.

I eventually accepted a faculty position at another university in Florida, earned tenure and promotion, and with funding support from the National Institutes of Health, I further developed the Talking Circle intervention and tested it within several randomized clinical trial studies among multiple Native American tribes in the United States and Indigenous populations globally using a community-based participatory research (CBPR) approach (Baldwin et al., 2020). These studies have yielded results that provided enough evidence that the Talking Circle was determined to be an evidence-based intervention. I also explored other ways to make an impact on the well-being of Native American people. For example, I collaborated with the late Dr. Roxanne Struthers to develop a nursing theoretical framework and model designed to guide nurses on how to provide culturally appropriate care to Native American people. The "Conceptual Framework of Nursing in Native American Culture" was first published in 2001 along with subsequent publications regarding how the framework can guide practice, management, and research (Lowe & Struthers, 2001; Lowe & Crow, 2009). With the vision to develop a center focused on Native American and Indigenous nursing research, I accepted a faculty position at yet another university in Florida, where I developed the Center for Indigenous Nursing Research for Health Equity, the first of its kind worldwide. Through the Center, I developed and hosted a summit where international Indigenous nurse researchers gathered to present and share the research that they were conducting among various Indigenous populations globally. These summits have continued, and the second one was held in Australia. Eventually, I left Florida and accepted a position at a research-intensive institution in Texas, where I am currently being supported to elevate research efforts to address health disparities and equity among Native American and Indigenous people in

> *The Talking Circle was determined to be an evidence-based intervention.*

the United States and globally along with preparing the next generation of Native/Indigenous nurse scientists. The third International Indigenous Nursing Research Summit is planned to be held in Texas.

Immersion Experiences

I observed how non-Native researchers would often come into Native American communities to conduct a research project on a topic/issue they identified as important and needing to be studied. After completing the project, the researcher most often disappeared, leaving nothing behind of benefit to the tribal community. I decided to develop a way to contribute and give back to tribal communities before, during, and after implementing a research project. Creating a strategy for nursing students to achieve learning objectives while immersed in tribal communities also provided those communities with unique health services. I developed a special tribal immersion program for senior RN-BSN nursing students to meet course objectives related to community health and transcultural nursing. The students, many who were from diverse cultures, traveled to Oklahoma from Florida and stayed within tribal communities to provide health services to tribal communities. Also, nursing students in the master's and doctoral programs were provided with opportunities to meet course objectives within the tribal communities by leading and providing various health programs. This created a way to intervene, while not conducting a funded intervention research project, by focusing on critical health issues such as diabetes, obesity, and substance abuse. The nursing students—many of whom are of international origin and hail from countries such as Cuba, Jamaica, and Haiti—stayed in the tribal communities and taught classes on nutrition, diabetes, and introduced various forms of physical activities in community schools, and summer camps. They also conducted health screenings and delivered presentations to tribal youth regarding disease prevention, health promotion, and career opportunities in health care. The students also shared information about the various cultures and countries of their origin, and they participated in traditional tribal events and ceremonies.

Providing health care to Native American people, as well as to other diverse and underserved populations, has become a popular focus among many healthcare disciplines. As a result, I am often sought after to provide guidance to those who would like to provide the "solution" and "answer" to health disparities, especially among Native Americans. My message has been simple but constant: Learn to become the learner. Many times, nurses and other healthcare professionals spend so much time becoming the "expert" that they forget they have much to learn from the diverse people they seek to provide care for. Nurses often learn to assess people and then tell them what's wrong with them and what they are going to do about it. Instead, learning from the person or community involves taking the approach of "you teach me," which can result in effective outcomes.

> *Learn to become the learner.*

Navigating Systems to Overcome Discrimination and Racism

In summary, my story is reflective of a journey with many rewarding achievements. At the same time, it has been a journey of confronting systems where discrimination and racism are embedded

in the infrastructure and fabric. In many ways, I was not prepared to navigate these systems, but I was fortified with a strong
Native American cultural identity and a deep knowing that I was
created for a purpose. Many of these systems were developed to
keep Native Americans out, and I have endured the intention of
being excluded and denied the privileges and rights others have
within those institutional systems. I have also experienced com-
plicit attempts within institutions to be professionally deterred,
destroyed, and eliminated from doing the important work to
address health disparities and promote health equity among Native
American and Indigenous people. Because of these experiences,
I am acutely aware of the discrimination and racism that continues to exist. The lessons learned from these experiences have deep-
ened my passion and motivation to prepare the next generation
of Native/Indigenous nurses to navigate systems so that they can
become healthcare leaders in research, education, and practice.

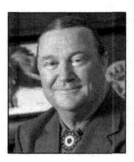

John Lowe, PhD, RN, FAAN

Dr. John Lowe is the Joseph Blades Centennial Memorial Professor at the University of Texas at Austin School of Nursing. He is a Cherokee Native American tribal member and also has Creek and Lenape Native American tribal heritage. Dr. Lowe currently serves as a member of the Advisory Council to the National Institutes of Nursing Research (NINR). He co-authored with Dr. Roxanne Struthers (Ojibwe) the Conceptual Framework for Nursing in Native American Culture. Dr. Lowe was the first Native American man to be inducted as a fellow in the American Academy of Nursing and currently serves as a member of the selection committee. He is an alumnus of the Minority Fellowship Program (MFP) at the American Nurses Association and has served as the chair of the National Advisory Council to the MFP. He developed and studies interventions for the prevention and reduction of substance use and other risk behaviors among Native American and Indigenous youth and young adults globally. These studies and other health programs are guided by models that Dr. Lowe developed, which include the Cherokee Self-Reliance, Native Self-Reliance, and Native-Reliance theoretical framework and models. Dr. Lowe also developed the first manualized Talking Circle intervention to reduce substance use and other risk behaviors among Native American/Indigenous youth in the United States and globally in countries such as Canada and Australia. His research projects have been funded by the National Institutes of Health, Substance Abuse and Mental Health Services Administration, and other organizations and foundations such as the Rita & Alex Hillman Foundation. The Talking Circle intervention has been recognized by the U.S. Department of Justice's Office of Justice Programs as a "Promising Evidence-Based Program" for the well-being of youth, recognized as the first manualized Talking Circle intervention, featured as one of the American Academy of Nursing's "Edge Runners," and most recently featured in the National Academy of Medicine report of *The Future of Nursing 2020–2030: Charting a Path to Achieve Health Equity*. He developed the first Center for Indigenous Nursing Research and hosted the first international Indigenous nursing research summit. Dr. Lowe's work also has been acknowledged through numerous awards such as the American Nurses Association Luther Christman Award, Florida Nurses Association Cultural Diversity Award, Great 100 Centennial Research Award, Nursing Educator of the Year Award, Nurse of the Year Award, Lifetime Achievement In Education & Research Award, and the Researcher of the Year at the Professor Rank Award. Dr. Lowe has presented nationally and internationally and has published several articles and books.

11

Breaking Barriers With Inclusiveness

Elizabeth McClure, DNP, MS, RN, NPD-BC

Why Did You Choose Nursing as a Career?

My family structure included being raised by grandparents and living in a community with extended family with old traditions. Success was measured by employment with the local wharfs, as it was a high-paying job without requiring college education. I always felt uncomfortable in school, as I was surrounded by schoolmates whose parents had professional careers and who lived in mid- to high-income communities. Throughout my school experience, I knew I wanted to have the same opportunities as my other classmates. I knew I wanted to have a meaningful life after high school; however, my parents were not clear on the process of attending college. Fortunately, my parents wanted me to break traditions and explore career options, which included attending a career fair in my local community. The memory of caring for my grandparents along with the struggles with language barrier, the attributes of the nursing profession was where I thought I could make an impact on other Hispanic people. I am very grateful for the support provided by my parents, as it was not an easy decision to go against family norms.

Describe Your Admission to a Nursing Program

The community college offered an associate degree (ADN) program with counselor guidance for admissions and financial support (i.e., scholarships). Completed high school courses did not meet the requirements for pre-nursing courses for the ADN program, which meant a year of college attendance prior to being an official student in the nursing program. The admission status opened the door to specific nursing scholarships, which reduced the number of part-time jobs I needed, and allowed me to focus more on completing the program.

Seven years after graduating from the ADN program, I completed my bachelor of nursing (BSN) degree program. During that time, I was working overseas at a hospital with many American expatriates. Fortunately, the Nursing Education and Research Center had nursing leadership that promoted higher education. The hospital agreed to jointly work with a university in the United States (U.S.) for a distance program. Due to military presence, University of Maryland was available where prerequisite courses could be taken to meet criteria for admissions. I was in the first cohort of nurses who decided to take the journey together in completing our BSN while continuing to work abroad. There were many more cohorts following our group, and as we were in our last year, the organization took another step in collaborating with another U.S. university for a distance master's program.

The same cohort for my BSN enrolled in the master's program; however, we took different paths (i.e., CNS, NP). University of Maryland was still available for any prerequisite courses if required. The admission criteria were no different than for any other student. The curriculum was designed where summer course attendance was required, and throughout the academic year courses were online, and clinicals required an approved preceptor. Accepting admission to the program, we knew it required traveling back to the U.S. to meet course and clinical expectations.

Pursuing a doctoral degree had not been an option since I was not able to justify the cost and time away from family obligations. However, as doctor of nursing practice (DNP) programs started to evolve and I had fewer family responsibilities, pursuing a DNP required further review. Gathering information through articles, speaking to others who had completed the program, and talking with the program director convinced me that it was time to proceed to the next milestone in my nursing career. My current employer had recently included the DNP program for tuition reimbursement, which made it difficult to pass on the opportunity. Meeting the admission criteria can be different for each student based on previous course completions. The most impactful part of the admission process included the interview, which really focused on your perception of the role of a DNP practitioner as well as your potential scholarly project. There was an emphasis on having an inclination toward a topic for your scholarly project. Of course, you were not committed to your initial project topic, but you were made aware of how changes could impact your progression toward expected graduation. Once all the course and clinical hours were finalized for meeting the admission criteria, the progression of the program was straightforward.

Progression and Challenges in the Program

Frequent challenges throughout the program were not being able to form consistent study groups or work on group projects due to work and/or family obligations. Development of consistent study habits led to succeeding in completion of the program. As I continued my advanced studies, the challenges flipped, as we had a core group of nurses who were committed to succeed. The hospital provided support in allowing time for study groups as well as resources from the nursing education and library department for support. Other considerations included having access to internet and computer technology, since the BSN and graduate school were overseas. The commitment from the organization made you feel that they wanted you to succeed.

The DNP program was fairly new, and the groups were not large, which made my experience in the program very positive as the faculty were accessible and just very supportive. The advances in technology provided a learning management system for students which made the experience more positive compared to previous nursing programs. Of course, technology has improved over the years, making it easier for a student to complete a program. Meeting classmates that worked in different healthcare institutions provided a network of resources postgraduation. Completing the DNP program was rewarding and the highest accomplishment in my nursing career. However, it was very disappointing to be asked what the degree meant among healthcare providers. I found it a great opportunity to encourage advanced nursing studies. Since my graduation 3 years ago, most of our educators within our department have either completed or are in progress to complete the DNP program.

Share About Your First Job and Your Career Progression

During nursing school, nurses from different specialties visited our nursing program, sharing their career experience. One of those was a flight nurse, which piqued my interest, but I knew that would be my future goal. I was fortunate that I had a nursing professor who reminded me that planning is essential to be successful. Therefore, I knew that I had to take every opportunity to succeed. My pre-nursing jobs included being an EKG technician and a companion in a nursing home for patients whose families lived out of town. Both pre-nursing jobs built my confidence in my social skills with patients and family members, which can be a huge hurdle to overcome as a young adult. As a senior nursing student, I accepted a nurse assistant (NA) job on a neurological/neurosurgical floor and worked along with senior RNs and LPNs.

My first journey as an RN continued on the unit where I had worked as an NA. Unfortunately, there was a misperception that since I had experience on that floor, I was ready to step in as a night charge nurse alongside an LPN. Of course, I thought this was normal and had to really depend on the LPN for guidance. As I look back on this experience, I do ask myself, "What was I thinking?" that this was okay. However, talking to other nurses and ex-classmates, we all faced the same scenario.

During my first year on the same unit, every opportunity was taken to attend ongoing education in caring for neurological patients. As patients from the neuro intensive care unit (ICU) were transferred to the floor, I was amazed with the knowledge and skills these nurses demonstrated. I knew that my new goal would be to be part of that team. After one year of floor experience, an opportunity arose to join the Neuro-ICU team, where over 90% of nurses were master's prepared. This was also a pivotal moment of my introduction to electronic patient documentation. The approach to orientation was like being back in school and included reading assignments and applying that knowledge to my current patient assignment. Patient rounds were led by the senior attending physician and included all interprofessional team members.

My goal to become a flight nurse remained on track. After 2 years of Neuro-ICU, hyperbaric and extracorporeal membrane oxygenator (ECMO) part-time positions, and a paramedic license, a position as a flight nurse opened, and I felt ready to apply. I remember talking to the head nurse about applying for the position, and her response was, "You will not get in since there are others with more experience." I was shocked and questioned myself about moving forward with the application. Fortunately, I had encouragement from other team members, including the neurosurgery physician team, which felt my experience would be an advantage in caring for neurotrauma patients. I finally met my goal and accepted the position as a flight nurse for 3 years.

> *The nursing profession allows you to meet different milestones.*

As you grow older, you find other interests, and I found myself wondering what was next for me. I had a German exchange student say to me, "You Americans have no idea what is going on in the world." A few days later, I met a nurse who had just returned from Saudi Arabia to attend the pediatric nurse practitioner program who shared her experience with me. Again, my interest was piqued!

The nursing profession allows you to meet different milestones. My new path now included traveling the world, which led me to a nursing job in Saudi Arabia. The nursing profession was not an acceptable career for the country; therefore, nurses were recruited from different countries to meet the nursing needs of the hospital. The expectation was that you practiced under your country's nursing licensure scope of practice. I was no longer that confident flight nurse as I faced language and cultural barriers from patients and coworkers.

Cultural and diversity workshops incorporated the "Culture Care Theory" in orientation as well as ongoing educational offerings throughout the year. Throughout the years, my position started as a staff nurse, I opened a training center for the American Heart Association's basic and advanced programs, and then I became manager for the emergency department. The Gulf War in 1990 was an unexpected challenge, with no avenue of leaving the country and a crash course on chemical warfare. This experience adjusted my lens through which I view the world, leading to respecting cultural diversity among patient care and nursing practices.

Academia became my next milestone while adjusting to living in America again. I now felt like a foreigner, as I had to readapt to day-to-day living, and I was anxious to see how much nursing practice might have changed while I was abroad. To my surprise, the equipment and standards of care were very similar to the practice in Saudi Arabia. However, teaching in academia was very different from a hospital setting. This was a great opportunity to apply my skills and knowledge from graduate school into the academic setting. My previous experience in the clinical setting as well as working with a diverse population provided me with strong skills in communicating with students from other countries. However, the emphasis on curriculum development was quite different from a staff development perspective. As I became more proficient in curriculum development, the transition to my next position in a hospital setting was more challenging.

My next and current journey is now as a nursing professional development (NPD) specialist. In this role, I am able to compare the differences between the academic and hospital setting. Most of the hospital's educators do not have a background in academia, so the thinking process is quite different. Preparing for the

> *My cumulative experience has been building blocks that have contributed to a wonderful journey in my nursing career.*

NPD certification provides an excellent framework for those in a hospital setting for planning educational activities. I do not think teaching in one setting is better than the other, as everyone has a part in contributing to someone's learning. My cumulative experience has been building blocks that have contributed to a wonderful journey in my nursing career.

Your Recommendations for Equity in the Future

You might have noticed that in the beginning I hinted that English was my second language. Throughout my nursing career, many had no idea that I am Hispanic. I was the first college graduate in my family and extended family. As I found nursing as a rewarding career, I made sure I met with high-school-aged relatives to provide some guidance postgraduation. Our family now has five Hispanic nurses. Relocating from the Middle East to the Midwest, there was not much diversity nor a well-known Hispanic community. That has changed over the years, with an increase in the Hispanic population for various reasons. Most recently, Hispanic nurses around the surrounding area have identified a need for a local National Association of Hispanic Nurses chapter addressing social determinants of health and promoting healthy environments. Membership is not limited to only nursing but other key stakeholders within the community as well.

Assessing our environment is a necessary process if equity is to be addressed to meet the evolving change in populations.

It's crucial to be aware of how foreign and domestic policy will impact your local community of a diverse population, short- and long-term. Providing culturally sensitive care for identified, targeted diverse populations should be considered when planning nursing professional development activities. Organizations should continue to have programs advertising and/or events promoting nursing and other healthcare careers in different venues targeting various age groups.

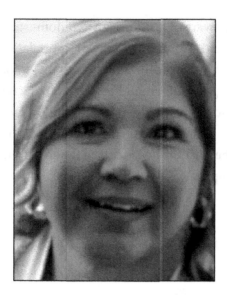

Elizabeth McClure, DNP, MS, RN, NPD-BC

Dr. McClure has been actively engaged in the practice of nursing for over 35 years, including 8 years in the Middle East in continuing education and clinical practice since 1985. In her current role, she is the accredited provider program director for Nursing Continuing Professional Development at St. Elizabeth Healthcare Organization and Development and maintains clinical practice at the University of Cincinnati Emergency Department. In addition, Dr. McClure has served 2 years as a volunteer on ANCC's Commission on Accreditation in Nursing Continuing Professional Development (COA-NCPD) as an emerging leader and currently representing the Healthcare Organization constituency. She is a member of several professional associations, including the American Nurses Association, Association for Nurses in Professional Development, and the Greater Cincinnati National Association of Hispanic Nurses.

12

From the Pearl of the Oriental Seas to Global Nursing Leadership

Cora Canlas-Munoz, PhD, RN

From the Pearl of the Orient Seas to the Skyscraper of New York City

Fifty years ago, as a new graduate from nursing school, I came to New York City from the Philippines. Every nurse in my country wanted to work abroad; however, I was not one of them. So, after obtaining my bachelor's degree from St. Paul University in Manila, I returned to my parents' home in the southern part of the country. I already had a new staff position at small private hospital, a job that my mother arranged with the physicians who owned this hospital. This was not unusual for my parents to use their connections to give me my first job. Eight months into this job, I started dreaming of going to the United States; not any state, but only to New York City. My attraction was the city of skyscrapers and the city that does not sleep, Broadway, bagels, and subways. I did not go through any travel agency, but I searched the U.S. hospitals looking for a job. I found the Foreign Exchange Nurses Visitors Program, and I applied. This was 1970. I was 22 years old. The trip to NYC was my first trip abroad. I was alone but very excited and felt so adventurous that I was not afraid or anxious at all. This was the beginning of my new life in the city that I had loved from afar.

Filipino Cultural Value on Education and Why I Chose Nursing as a Career

I came from a family of educators. My mother was a science teacher and guidance counselor, and my father was a certified public accountant. They had eight children, all eight children graduated college, six earned a master's degree, and three of the eight siblings earned a PhD. One became a president of a college in Southern Philippines and was a visiting professor at The Ohio State University, where he completed his PhD. Another became a secretary of education in the Philippines and a vice president of the University of the East where she graduated, and then she retired as the executive director of Southeast Asian Innovation Technology and earned a PhD. Currently, she is the president of a polytechnic institute in the Philippines. Other siblings have a master's in business and finance and taught real estate management at a community college, a master's in sociology and was a professor at a state university in Southern Philippines, a master's in dietetics and was involved in patient education and training. We are a family of educators.

This was exactly why I wanted to be a nurse: to help those who are not able to care for themselves because of illness.

So why did I choose nursing? This was not a welcomed idea for a profession. It was implied in my family that the best and most secure career for a female with job security is to go into education. I was quite young when I knew that I wanted to be a nurse. We had no family member in the medical profession, yet I wanted to be able to take care of the sick and help families handle the challenge of having a sick member of their family. My father was strongly against my career choice because he wanted to spare me from the "hard and dirty" work that nurses need to do for others. This was exactly why I wanted to be a nurse: to help those who are not able to care for themselves because of illness. I wanted to serve others who are sick—the weak and the vulnerable. My mother used to remind me that as a child, I was first to respond to anyone in the family who was hurt and needed to tend to cuts and bruises. My mother knew that caring for others is what I would do when I grew up.

Since my parents were financially fully supporting me to go to college, I complied with my father's suggestion not to be a nurse. So, in the first year of college, I matriculated as an undecided major taking general courses because I knew that I would eventually switch to nursing as my major. True enough, after one year of taking liberal arts courses, I switched to nursing. I convinced my family that I was up to the hard work of becoming a nurse and that there is job security in this profession. This was the best decision I have made in my life and have totally no regrets. The nursing program was rigid and demanding. The bachelor's degree in nursing was a 5-year study at that time for a full-time student in this program. I went to an all-girls, private Catholic college of nursing with a high rating for success in the national nursing licensure exam. My father was absolutely right in that nursing is hard and we have to do some of the dirty work involved in providing physical care for patients.

Admission to St. Paul University in Manila

I was admitted to the nursing program at St. Paul University in Manila, Philippines. This is an all-girls private Catholic institution.

It is a highly selective admission process not only academically but also since it is a private institution, the tuition fees were higher than other schools, particularly compared to government-run or city-owned schools of nursing. My admission to the program was uneventful other than the tuition fees that became a burden to my parents, who continued to support me fully for 5 years. Working while in school was not an acceptable option. My parents worked hard to send all their 8 children to college.

Progression and Challenges in the Nursing Program

I progressed well in the nursing program. We were a cohort of over 100 in a class, and about one third graduated in 5 years. We were constantly reminded that passing the nursing licensure exam brings much credibility to the program and to the school and therefore failing a nursing licensure exam was not an option. This was a daily and constant reminder that was quite stressful for any student. Additionally, we were strongly encouraged to pursue graduate studies and told that obtaining a bachelor of science in nursing is not the terminal degree. Today, I am one of three in my class who pursued a doctoral degree in nursing, and several have master's degrees as well.

Clinical experience in the hospital was every day starting at 6 a.m. until noon. Then at 1 p.m., we attended academic classes as a cohort until 5 p.m. We had a brief time to grab lunch and switch from the white clinical uniform with white nursing shoes and white nursing cap to the university school uniform of black checkered skirt and white long sleeve shirt with a black tie and a college pin and black pumps. This was required campus attire as stated in the nursing uniform code and university policy. We were not allowed to wear clinical attire to the classroom setting, the rationale being that there may be contaminants in the clinical uniform that could spread to the classroom. This Catholic nun-run school had very strict and rigid rules that personally became challenging for me, and it became very difficult to comply unless I was convinced of their rationale. I often debated and challenged the nuns to explain the thinking behind a rule or a policy. I was not in their list of "favorite" or "compliant" students.

One of the big challenges was the hectic schedule with packed clinical hours to complete. Clinical placement included operating room rotation as a circulating nurse, hospital kitchen experience for therapeutic dietetics, and others that I thought were not necessary in the basic nursing curriculum. We were required to take several courses in theology as well as a course in social graces, with which I constantly disagreed as a requirement rather than an elective. Overall, I did well with my nursing and liberal arts courses, including those courses I resented to take but had to.

First Job and Career Progression in America

My first job after graduation was at a small private hospital in Southern Philippines, a 20-bed private hospital owned by a group of physicians. As a staff nurse in my first year after graduation, I was responsible for the entire patient population, including the nursery, emergency department, and emergency surgeries. It was extremely overwhelming to say the least. A night shift would be comprised of one RN and two aides. A physician was on call, as well as the head nurse/supervisor who occasionally needed to help in emergency clinical situations. I was frequently asked what a new graduate nurse was doing in a small hospital in the province with a meager salary instead of working abroad with an enticing pay scale and exciting new place in a foreign country. As mentioned before, working abroad was not in my career trajectory; however, after several months had passed, I was considering moving back to the big city and working in a metropolitan hospital. However, my parents were not supportive of this plan. Essentially, I was told that I needed to stay home and work in a local hospital unless I was planning to travel abroad. I immediately entertained the idea of employment in a foreign country. I was accepted into the Foreign Exchange Nurses Visitors Program at Columbia Presbyterian Hospital. The flight to New York City took 2 days with an overnight layover in Hong Kong from the Philippines. I was excited to be in a new country with a lot of possibilities for professional growth and personal development. I realized I was alone in a new place but ready to meet new people. I knew there are no strangers in this world because they are just friends whom we have not yet met. I was open to learn and explore!

It was the first time that I worked with many nurses from different countries. The Foreign Exchange Nurses Visitors Program was developed in response to the nursing shortage in the United States (Masselink & Jones, 2014). Filipino nurses were particularly interested in this program, and because English was the medium of instruction in the Philippines and the second official language of the country, language was not a barrier to employment in the United States. There were about 18 foreign exchange nurses in the program at Columbia Presbyterian Hospital. Countries represented in my class were Israel, Japan, Taiwan, India, the Philippines, Sweden, Denmark, Australia, Spain, the Netherlands, and China.

The program was designed to introduce the foreign exchange nurse to the nursing system and delivery of health care in the United States as well as provide educational experiences on the history of the United States and other sociocultural activities. We had history classes that included the history of slavery and oppression experienced by Black Americans. In the museum, we learned about natural history and the artistic display of work of U.S. artists. One of the highlights of this program was a visit to the home of nurse leader, author, and theorist Virginia Henderson in Upstate New York by the Hudson. I was in awe of the fact that someone with prominence in nursing met with us, and we had a wonderful exchange of ideas about nursing in our respective countries. Virginia Henderson was so engaging and so personable.

We also had experiences working as staff nurses, though not licensed in NYC. We were providing care under the supervision and preceptorship of a registered nurse. Caring is indeed universal, so nursing care was easy for us to provide. The technology was new to most of us, but we were interested, excited, and quick to learn. In the meantime, we were also learning about each other in the class, which was very diverse in countries of origin. We did cultural presentations for each other and appreciated the cultural beliefs, practices, and perspectives that were different. Cultural sensitivity and cultural humility indeed were operative then. This must be the first time I started to look at individuals with acceptance and respect of the differences and what they bring that enhances relationships. Friendships started, and our relationships were crystallized for 12 months in the program.

We all worked and played together, traveled to many cities in the country, and explored thoroughly what New York City had to offer. I was finally in the city that never sleeps. As international students, we were invited to opening nights at Broadway and the Metropolitan Opera at Lincoln Center. Baryshnikov and Nureyev, the NY Philharmonic, and the Jeoffrey Ballet were some of the performances we saw with free or discounted tickets on opening week for the press to review and critique the shows. We were so fortunate and so blessed! It was so much fun!

As we enjoyed the city, we were warned to keep safe and be careful walking the streets of New York City. I was perplexed when we were told that whenever we saw a group of Black teens coming our way, we should cross to the other side of the street and by all means avoid them and do not make eye contact with them. Having no preconceived ideas about Black people in America and not understanding the historical context of this comment, this warning was something that disturbed me for a long time. Several months later, when I was working as a staff nurse, I found myself on the subway at the crack of dawn to start my 7 a.m. shift, and sitting across from me were 5 young Black teens in an otherwise empty subway car. One of them got up to sit next to me. Immediately, the warning rose to my consciousness, though I was not afraid. I spoke first to tell them with direct eye contact that I was a nurse (wearing my white uniform and white shoes, carrying my nurses cap in a zippered plastic pocket) and that I was going to work for a morning shift. The young Black teen sitting next to me said in a perplexed voice, "Are you not afraid of us?" to which I replied, "Should I be afraid of you?" Tension dropped, and he said most people are afraid when they see a group of Black teens coming their way. He continued to say, "We will not hurt anybody." I said, "I know you will not." In my heart, I knew that I had just dispelled a bias that is destructive against a group of people.

Neurological Institute: Diverse Patient Population

Columbia Presbyterian Hospital is a metropolitan hospital with over 2,500 hospital beds. When the Foreign Exchange Nurse Visiting Program ended, about half in my class applied for an immigrant visa and therefore we were able to work as staff nurses at the medical center. I worked in a general surgical unit for several

months and then took a staff nurse position in the neurological intensive care unit (Neuro-ICU) at the Neurological Institute,
one of the ten hospitals at Columbia Presbyterian Medical Center.
This position was very demanding but professionally very rewarding. As a teaching hospital, we all continued to learn from the physicians and surgeons, from nurses, and all auxiliary professionals.
The patients were very diverse, primarily Caucasian, African American, and Hispanic/Latino. However, the staff was predominantly
White. I observed early on that the care provided for these patients
did not seem to take into consideration their cultural and ethnic
backgrounds. There were no interpreters, and families served to
address the language barriers. Health disparities in the early 70s
had not been widely addressed in the literature or in clinical practice. I knew that all patients needed to be treated with respect,
and they all deserved to receive equal treatment of the best quality care. I also knew that there was structural racism in the healthcare system in the United States and that people of color do receive
unequal treatment and have a disproportionate incidence of mortality and morbidity. Healthcare providers unknowingly contribute
to this disparity. Implicit biases negatively impact clinical decisions
in patient care, and this leads to poor quality of care and patient
dissatisfaction. In the early 70s and 80s, attention to this matter was
not a priority, although health disparities did exist.

I requested a transfer from the Neuro-ICU to the Neuropsychiatric unit in the same hospital building. This was a 12-bed locked
unit on the 12th floor of the Neurological Institute. I wanted a less
routine type of nursing care. I knew that those patients with neurological and/or psychiatric disorders would be more challenging and much less routine work. Behaviors are so individually
expressed and are greatly influenced by one's cultural background,
and this was exciting to me. The psychiatrists at that time were

also expected to train as neurologists. This seemed to be a precursor of the Decade of the Brain from 1990 to 2000, during which the National Institutes of Health (NIH) focused on exploring the brain, particularly on understanding brain disorders such as Parkinson's disease and Alzheimer's disease that had been debilitating for millions of Americans and were very costly to treat (Library of Congress, n.d.).

During the Decade of the Brain, I had an opportunity to be invited for an NIH training. It was mind-boggling to me. I was so amazed with the use of technology and new brain imaging, revealing new scientific breakthroughs. This was the highlight of my nursing career at that time—having information that was cutting edge based on current research and an explosion of new therapeutics for patients with neurologic and psychiatric disorders. Now, mental illness has been relabeled as the disease of the mind and of the brain. I hoped stigmatization of mental disorders would diminish, but unfortunately, stigmatization continued. Cultural definitions of illness and health such as mental health vary from group to group.

The Neurological and Psychiatric Unit

From staff nurse at this neuropsychiatric unit, I eventually became an assistant nurse manager, and then in a couple of years I was promoted to nurse manager (then referred to as head nurse). I worked with wonderful neuropsychiatrists and neuropsychiatric nurses. They were my mentors. They treated me with respect and appreciation of what I brought to the team in terms of knowledge, skills, leadership, and quality nursing care. I was the only Asian nurse manager in this unit. I worked with only one Filipino nurse in psychiatric mental health, who became a very close friend to this day. She is a gem! Filipino nurses generally shun psychiatric nursing, and most of them work in medical–surgical units and intensive care units. Here, nursing care primarily involves tasks, whereas in psychiatric mental health settings, nursing care is primarily focused on therapeutic communications, interpersonal skills, and behavioral interventions. Being clear, articulate, and precise in language is expected of a psychiatric nurse in addition to astute observations of behaviors. I was in this unit for many years. I felt confident as I gained expertise and specialization as a psychiatric mental health nurse. I knew my therapeutic interaction skills and the nursing process, as well as psychopharmacologic interventions.

My performance evaluations were all very good to outstanding. In one of the earlier evaluations, after I was given very positive feedback on my clinical performance, the nurse manager told me, "Cora, your long, straight black hair makes you look very oriental." After she stated this and I signed the evaluation, she left the room. I was flabbergasted! Why did she say that? Why did I not ask what she was trying to say or meant to say? Why did she leave the room right away? What was wrong with having long black hair? What was wrong with looking Asian, which I am? What messages was she wanting me to receive? These were the questions in my mind that came in rather quick succession. I was still wondering what this was about. After reading up on cultural differences, I realized the context of her comment was the melting pot theory that was operative in the 70s and 80s in America. The goal of the melting pot theory is to minimize and diminish differences so everyone in America would look more alike than different (American History Today, n.d.). Being different can be intimidating and threatening. I decided to cut my hair short and changed my hair color from black to brown. The melting pot theory did not work, because it is not possible to change physical appearance and the color of one's skin. Additionally, the melting pot theory discredits and devalues what immigrants bring to this country. In fact, immigrants have contributed valuable resources to society that enriched America to become the multicultural nation that it is. What is operative now is an appreciation of diversity and unity, and the ultimate goal is equity for all. This country is still quite far from achieving this goal.

> *The melting pot theory discredits and devalues what immigrants bring to this country. In fact, immigrants have contributed valuable resources to society that enriched America to become the multicultural nation that it is.*

As a nurse manager of the neuropsychiatric unit, I was invited to attend one of the American Psychiatric Association meetings on the *Diagnostic and Statistical Manual of Mental Disorders* (*DSM-I*) at the Psychiatric Institute, representing the medical director of the neuropsychiatric unit, with whom I worked closely. This was a small group of psychiatrists, all older White men making decisions on the nomenclature of mental illness that would be used across the country. It was rather intimidating for me to be at the meeting. I was a young, female registered nurse of Asian descent among these older White male psychiatrists. Immediately, I wondered how this group could even begin to appreciate and understand the role of culture and ethnicity in diagnosing mental illness. The melting pot theory was operative at that time; however, the mental healthcare system still operated on a Eurocentric perspective. Racism, discrimination, and prejudices were already experienced by patients and families and in the larger society, but these issues were generally ignored or minimized. Little was known as to their impact on physical and mental health. The literature at that time already had identified health disparities in mental health, particularly the problem with misdiagnosis of schizophrenia in African Americans. Clearly there was limited consideration and understanding of the role of culture in understanding behaviors and in diagnosing mental illness. Again, note that the guide for diagnosis was developed and designed for the most part by White older male mental health professionals. Behaviors and thoughts are so greatly influenced by one's cultural experiences and socialization.

Graduate Education at Columbia University

It was only when I moved to New York City and worked at a large medical center that I noticed the very diverse patient population. Columbia Presbyterian Medical Center is in Washington Heights in Uptown Manhattan. The client population was primarily Hispanic and African American and some Asian patients. The diversity was new to me compared to the population in the Philippines where I am originally from. Based on my clinical observations, I concluded that Hispanic and Black patients were not provided equitable quality care. No interpreters were generally available at that time. Clearly this negatively impacts healthcare outcomes and quality care.

I worked on my master's degree in teaching nursing at Columbia University Teachers College. As staff at the medical center, I received full tuition reimbursement for Columbia University, a private Ivy League institution. I had only one minority faculty in my entire nursing master's program. I felt compelled to go to graduate school; after all, this was my family's expectation and a highly valued practice. Columbia University is a private institution, tuition was free, and the quality of education is exemplary. Who would want to bypass this educational opportunity? I now have a formal background in teaching, and like my mother and my siblings, I have become an educator. Since my graduate degree is in nursing education, being a teacher was my primary role in the classroom and clinical practice.

I quickly realized that teaching was not only very rewarding but I also felt that the impact of one good, caring, competent, and humanistic nurse educator upon the nursing students she teaches is priceless. The Johnson & Johnson campaign to increase interest in the nursing profession depicted this sentiment in the portrayal of one nurse educator who touches the lives of so many students and therefore, in essence, is present in the day-to-day nursing care provided by those who learned the science and art of nursing from the caring teacher (Johnson & Johnson, 2016). Later, I dwelled on the idea that the nurse educator really contributes significantly to the cognitive, social, educational, spiritual, and cultural learning dimensions of the student. The nurse educator molds the hearts of the learner to be caring and compassionate, stimulating their critical thinking skills for sound and evidence-based clinical judgments and weaving a moral, spiritual, and ethical fabric that all patients deserve the best nursing care regardless of race, creed, cultural background, and ethnicity. Indeed, every person needing nursing care needs to be provided with the highest quality of care. This is acknowledging human dignity and promoting social justice for all.

Teaching Nursing

My first teaching job was at the McConnell Clark School of Nursing at Columbia Presbyterian Medical Center. This is an associate degree in nursing (ADN) program that had a very diverse student population as well as diverse faculty and staff. It attracted those with a degree and license in practical nursing for upward educational mobility that leads to an associate degree and licensure as a registered nurse. A lot of the students were older with families to take care of, and some had a job in addition to being a full-time student. As faculty, we were very cognizant of these multiple roles that increased stress on the students. As previously indicated, teaching is so rewarding and satisfying, knowing that one has a role in preparing professionals whose practice will make a difference in the lives of so many patients and families they interact with.

My teaching load was both didactic/theoretical and in clinical practice. I was teaching psychiatric mental health nursing, and for clinical placement we used the neuropsychiatric (Neuro12) unit at Neurological Institute of Columbia Presbyterian Medical Center and at New York Psychiatric Institute (PI), a state mental hospital. The hospitals were adjacent to each other, so I was doing clinical supervision for my clinical group split between Neuro12 and PI. For the first time, I experienced the health disparities with racial and ethnic minority patients in the mental health system. I had read in professional literature about the issue of misdiagnosis of Black psychiatric patients. I observed this on many occasions when my students took care of White patients at the Neuro12 unit and Black patients at the Psychiatric Institute, demonstrating similar psychiatric symptomatology but given different diagnoses. The Black patient would typically be diagnosed with schizophrenia and the White patient diagnosed with an affective disorder. It was quite disturbing to know the serious implications of having a diagnosis of schizophrenia on the Black patient. It had severe negative impact on the lives of the Black patients in terms of treatment options and the stigma associated with the diagnosis.

We had another case that I will always remember in terms of cultural sensitivity and culturally competent care in psychiatric mental health. My student was working with an adolescent female from one of the Caribbean islands. She was admitted to the adolescent unit of the Psychiatric Institute for a severe psychotic break. Her mother brought her in for treatment of disturbing and distressing behavior of delusions and hallucinations. The patient was extremely fearful and out of touch with reality. The treatment team included psychopharmacologic interventions in the plan of care for psychosis. For several weeks, the psychosis did not diminish, and the patient increasingly became agitated with continued distorted experiences. Seeking a better understanding of the family dynamics and what happened prior to this psychotic break, the treatment team decided to seek the mother's perspective and invited her to the treatment team meeting about the case of her daughter. When asked what she thought caused this problem with her adolescent child, she replied with firm confidence and without hesitation that she believed her daughter was hexed. Everyone in the room was quiet and seemed surprised and shocked to hear the mother's explanation. The responses from the mother clearly indicated a belief in the magico-religious explanation of illness that is so different from the scientifically based Western explanation of mental illness that the professionals subscribed to. Clearly a conflict existed between the professional paradigm and the lay person/community perspective. Acknowledging that antipsychotic medications were not helping the patient in terms of alleviating emotional distress, the team again solicited the mother's help. What did she think could help her daughter and who did she think could help her daughter? She replied that she recommended a community healer to carry out a ritual to un-hex her daughter. Again, the treatment team was shocked and surprised; however, there was agreement that it was worth trying if the ritual was moral, ethical, legal, and not destructive to anyone or anything. Two weeks after the ritual was carried out, the patient showed dramatic improvement in psychotic symptoms. Overall, the treatment team agreed that culturally competent care was the key to this positive outcome. It took time and acknowledgment of cultural beliefs and practices with cultural humility that led to the improvement of the patient. After all, this is what every healthcare provider wanted as an outcome.

I later decided to pursue another graduate degree, so I matriculated at Hunter College in their master's in science program in psychiatric mental health nursing. My study was interrupted by the early death of my husband, Jaime Munoz. He was a lawyer, working in New York City, healthy and had a vibrant life. Unfortunately, as a smoker since his teenage years, he succumbed to cancer of the lungs.

Personal Challenge

After being married for 4 years with two young children, ages 2½ and 2 months, my husband passed away after 2 months from diagnosis to death. This was a serious personal tragedy. When my husband was admitted into the oncology unit of Columbia Presbyterian Medical Center, I was in the labor and delivery room having our second child at the same time at the same hospital. I was discharged after a week post-Cesarean delivery, and he remained in the hospital for 2 months until his death. As a single parent in the city that I love, I was at a crossroads as to how I could manage taking care of my two young children with good friends in New York City but with no family around for support. So, with much prayer for guidance and discernment, I decided to move to Columbus, Ohio, where most of my family live. This was one of the best decisions I have ever made in life. I had my extended family for support, especially during my first year of bereavement. All was possible because of God who gave me strength and hope.

From Manhattan to Columbus, Ohio

I decided to take the Holmes-Rahe inventory for stress level predicting the effect of stress on an individual (American Institute of Stress, n.d.). My stress level was over 450. The points added were the following: death of a spouse, new house, new job, new baby, new school for children, and new driving skill (I learned how to drive only after my husband passed away). I was in a very heightened stress level. With my score of 450, it is predicted that the person will end up needing hospitalization. Fortunately, I had good coping skills, family around for support, and a strong, solid spiritual foundation as a Catholic believing that God has a plan for all of us. We may not understand it now, but God's plan is always for good. As we go through life's trials and tribulations, God is always with us, and He will never abandon us, especially in time of need.

I interviewed for teaching jobs in Columbus, and each time after an interview, I was offered a job. This was encouraging for me to know that I could find work rather easily. I decided to accept a position as assistant professor at Ohio Wesleyan University (OWU). This is a private liberal arts university in Delaware, Ohio, considered by U.S. News and World Report to be one of the top 100 "Best National Liberal Arts Colleges" (U.S. News and World Report, n.d.). I was so excited to visit campus for the first time. The student population was predominately White and so were the faculty and staff. I surely added diversity to their faculty but later was told that they were impressed primarily with my degree from Columbia University and my clinical and teaching experience in New York City. The nursing department was fairly new, with a reputation for academic excellence. I taught psychiatric mental health nursing and community health. I eventually was tenured through a tenure committee that was supportive of professional programs. It was a wonderful experience teaching both in the classroom and in the clinical setting. I continued to be affirmed that teaching nursing was my calling, as I thoroughly enjoyed working with students and being instrumental in helping them develop the values and practices of a professional nurse. The rewards kept on coming in ways that were surprising. I heard from my former students and their parents thanking me for how I had impacted the lives of the student. Some of my former students are now my faculty colleagues, and I am so proud of them. They remind me that I made a difference in their professional journey as a nurse. I really believe it is a gift that keeps on giving in many ways. How wonderful it is to be a nurse educator! Joy is not from the monetary compensation but in one's role in making a difference and the impact on the lives of those learners who crossed your path in education.

At that time in 1983, culture and diversity were not much integrated into the nursing program, although the demographics of the country had started to change. In 1988, I attended a cultural competency presentation at The Ohio State University and met one of the trailblazers in transcultural nursing who was the presenter. I attribute my interest and passion in this subject area to her expertise and work in publications and presentations. I consider her my mentor and my friend. To this day, I continue to follow her footsteps. I am a transcultural care specialist, consultant, trainer, author, and scholar—all inspired by my dear mentor and friend!

After 12 years teaching at OWU, the faculty, which is predominantly White men, recommended to the board to phase out the nursing program that was an all-female faculty. I was one of the faculty selected to teach until the last class graduated. The dean of the nursing program was very supportive of me all throughout my time at OWU and during the final phase-out period. As one of the faculty who continued until the program was phased out, we were given a generous severance package including all the benefits of a faculty member, such as full tuition benefits for dependents. My son, Carlo, graduated from OWU in the journalism department and is currently working as a journalist with expertise in the military in Washington, DC.

Doctoral Program at The Ohio State University

When I was married, I decided to focus on my family and not pursue any post-master's degree. The plan was for me to work part time and live in Westchester County in New York. My life and my life's plan were totally changed when my husband passed away at 45 years old.

While at OWU, I knew that the only way to find a secure future in academia was to pursue a PhD. This was not in my plan, and I emotionally resisted the idea. However, the reality pointed to going back to school to have job security. I knew that teaching was now my path, and clearly I was moving into my career trajectory. As a doctoral student, I experienced the best learning in my life. My major was counselor education, and my minor was nursing education. I took several courses on diversity and cultural competency and cultural anthropology. My interest in this area became more and more deep and I was committed to increasing my knowledge about cultural sensitivity and health disparities.

While in school, I was working full time with 2 children to care for. I am blessed with my mother, who became my partner in managing my home and in the care of my children, along with a nanny who lived with us who alleviated my stress, especially after long days at work and evening classes. My children now are married with children. Carlo is a journalist in DC and Erica is a social worker with license master's in social work (LMSW) in New York City.

Professional Challenges and Inequity in Academia

When I earned my PhD degree, I accepted a tenure track position as an associate professor in nursing at Capital University in Columbus, Ohio. I continued to teach psychiatric mental health nursing for undergraduates and education courses at the graduate level. The student population is predominantly White, though its goal is to serve a diverse population. The faculty is increasingly diverse; however, the nursing faculty continues to be predominately female and White.

The first year I was at Capital University, there was an incident where a Black male professor's office door was vandalized with a sign blocked across it: "A N— teaches here." I was the only Asian faculty in the nursing department at that time. This was the first time that I had heard about a blatant and outright racist gesture made toward any faculty by students on campus. This Black colleague who was racially attacked was an outstanding faculty member and had received the highest award for teaching. Being new to my teaching job at the time, I do not know how this racism was addressed by the university administration. Years later, the victimized Black faculty member left the university. This was a profound loss for the department and for the entire university, and especially a loss for the students; he was an outstanding educator. I knew that racism destroyed lives every day.

> *I knew that racism destroyed lives every day.*

I had not overtly experienced any discrimination or prejudice during my entire time in New York City as a nurse and faculty member. I may not have been picking up on microaggressions as they exist today. All I knew was that I must work 200% harder than my counterparts to be able to achieve my professional goals and excel in my professional work. So, I worked 200% to get my promotion and tenure. When the time came for me to apply for tenure, I was informally discouraged to do so by the nursing administrator and was warned that it may not be the right time. There were two nursing faculty members up for tenure review, and we were both invited to a meeting with the university provost, directly discouraging us to apply for tenure. This seemed so unfair, and perhaps illegal, when the two of us followed tenure process criteria. I knew that I had met all the criteria for tenure and beyond. My teaching, scholarship, and community service were outstanding and more. I knew that I followed all the correct processes and procedures and that if I was denied tenure, it would lead to a case on discriminatory and unfair practice. My colleague did not want to proceed because it was better to leave the university before tenure was denied, as it would have a negative impact on future employment in academia. She resigned; I applied for tenure and got it.

I continue to teach in the graduate, undergraduate, BSN completion, and nursing accelerated programs at Capital University. I actively participated in college and university committees. I was honored to be invited and recommended by the dean to participate in a newly formed university committee to address accreditation issues. A newly hired assistant provost chaired this committee, which included faculty selected from the various disciplines. This was important work since the Higher Learning Commission had several conditions that needed to be addressed. My selection to this committee was questioned by another faculty member. She told me that the reason I was selected was because the new vice provost, hired from New York City with expertise and high credibility in accreditation, was Asian. Wow! This was a blatant microaggression!!! What a racist comment! This faculty member was known to be sensitive to cultural needs of students and had been working closely with non-White international students. She was a psychiatric nurse, and we had worked very closely for many years. She was a tenured faculty but did not have a doctoral degree. I was not able to react and respond as quickly as I wanted. My initial reaction was shock. My first thought was perhaps she wished she was selected instead of me. Later, and through the years, I became convinced that it was a racist remark—a microaggression toward me. I did not allow this to bother me, since I could recite my academic qualifications and eligibility to deserve such a selection. The committee work was long and demanding but was very productive and rewarding. I did not dwell on this. In the meantime, I accepted the reality that there is racism in academia to this day.

I sought faculty at Capital University who were champions for equity and cultural competence for our students. We advocated for students to appreciate culture and respect differences. In the student program outcome, we were able to include a statement indicating that we believe that graduates from Capital University are prepared to work in a diverse workforce in society. Working with faculty from the education and social work departments, we received a grant to be trained in multicultural communications in Portland, Oregon, at the Intercultural Institute. Additionally, we developed a course on Multidisciplinary Cultural Competence for the Helping Professionals. This was an interdisciplinary course offered to nursing, education, and social work students. This also was shared in peer-reviewed journals and national conferences.

> *I accepted the reality that there is racism in academia to this day.*

Opportunities

For many years, I was teaching a course on transcultural nursing in the undergraduate and the BSN completion programs at Capital. This continued post-retirement as adjunct faculty at Capital University and Mount Carmel College of Nursing. Additionally, I have been a consultant and trainer on cultural competency since the mid-80s. Today, I continue to do presentations, webinars, workshops, and seminars on culture and health for healthcare providers, physicians, nurses, social workers, counselors, mental health advocates, hospital staff, and government health agencies.

The university supported a lot of my educational travels to Sweden, China, Peru, Thailand, the Philippines, Australia, New Zealand, Finland, Denmark, Russia, the United Kingdom, and the Caribbean. I did scholarly presentations mainly on cultural competency, psychiatric mental health nursing, transcultural nursing, and teaching strategies and curriculum development.

I was also blessed and fortunate to be accepted as a Fulbright scholar in the specialist program three times. The focus of the Fulbright visit has primarily been global health and professional faculty development for nurse educators. This was a competitive application for educators, not necessarily in nursing, to be ambassadors representing the State Department of the United States to countries needing assistance in education. These three Fulbright scholarships were the highlight of my professional career as a nurse educator. These experiences led to establishing international partnerships with Capital University, China, and Thailand schools of nursing.

My desire to advocate for the vulnerable and marginalized populations experiencing health disparities and inequity is more intense than ever before. This is partly due to the sociopolitical climate of this country and the advent of the COVID-19 pandemic that brought attention to the existing health disparities in communities of color. It is time to fully address and eliminate health disparities in minority populations.

For so long, the social determinants of health have not been in the forefront of healthcare delivery and access. We know that social determinants of health explain a significant number of the causes of health problems. We must examine the broader factors that contribute to health disparities, such as the environment, safety, employment, housing, food availability, and access to transportation. Where we live determines how long we will live. Advocating for health equity is a matter of life and death. Every person in this nation deserves to receive care that is equitable and of the highest quality. This is an issue of social justice, equity, and respect for human dignity and rights. I strongly believe that everyone in the healthcare and helping professions must understand how social determinants of health impact and are impacted by culture and ethnicity. This needs to be integrated into the healthcare curriculum.

> *Where we live determines how long we will live. Advocating for health equity is a matter of life and death.*

During the COVID-19 pandemic, I had several opportunities to serve and be involved in advocacy efforts for communities of color. With my experience and expertise serving in the Ohio Commission on Minority Health for almost 20 years, the Ohio governor appointed me to be part of the Minority Health Strike Force to address health disparities and promote health equity for minority populations in Ohio. This statewide selected committee produced a report and specific recommendations primarily to address the disproportionate incidence of morbidity and mortality related to COVID-19. As a result, it also revealed the long-standing health disparities (Health Policy Institute of Ohio, 2020).

I have been part of numerous community initiatives to help in the COVID-19 testing, vaccination education, and vaccination campaign, particularly in Asian communities. Cultural and linguistic barriers needed to be addressed in planning services for this community. Dispelling beliefs and negative information about vaccination is challenging due to cultural nuances and linguistic issues. I also served as an expert panelist in the Ohio COVID-19 statewide needs assessment, producing a report identifying specific issues related to minority populations during the pandemic, in which specific recommendations were identified (The Ohio State University College of Public Health, 2020).

Work Continues to Achieve Health Equity

I earned emeritus status in 2011 when I retired from the Capital University School of Nursing. The semester immediately following my retirement, I accepted an adjunct position to teach transcultural nursing and graduate courses in the nursing education concentration.

I have been involved in community health initiatives providing comprehensive health screenings and education to the public to help alleviate disparities due to lack of access to health care. Support through grants from the county and other private foundations allows us to provide much-needed education during this pandemic. As president of the Ohio Asian American Health Coalition, I lead numerous initiatives to meet the unique needs of Asian communities, including civic engagement, mental health, and prevalent physical health disorders such as Hepatitis B, cardiovascular and respiratory problems, and diabetes. The current issue of anti-Asian violence and hate has been disturbing, particularly on the east and west coasts of the country. Though this is not new, the situation is alarming and unacceptable.

I have served for many years as a governor-appointed member of the Ohio Advisory Council to the Governor on AAPI Affairs and appointed to the Minority Health Vaccine Team of the Ohio Department of Health. I currently serve on the Franklin County Public Health Equity Advisory Board, HealthMap 2022 Steering Committee, vice-chair of the Ohio Institute of Communities of Color, OSU Cancer Community Advisory Board, president of the Asian Festival Corporation, and chair of the Asian Physician Advisory Group, among many other boards.

I believe in giving back to the profession and the community at large after gaining the wealth of experience and expertise in nursing as a profession and in education. I have been involved in nursing practice and teaching nursing for almost 52 years and have much to share with the next generation. I have mentored many individuals and would like to share comments from an interview with one of my mentees, who has become a special nursing leader:

> When I asked her about the differences with the challenges when she first started her career versus today, Dr. Munoz said, "It certainly is very different today. Nursing practice has evolved to become a profession, in that our clinical judgments are based on evidence. Use of technology has become the norm, and there are certain advantages to that, such as electronic medical records and care equipment are more precise. What is important is for nurses to remember that nursing care is a science as well as an art. Therefore,

the humanistic aspect must be intentional and deliberate in planning care that also includes therapeutic touch and cultural sensitivity and cultural competence."

When asked about what advice to give to the younger generation of nurses, she stated, "Practice your profession that is grounded on evidence but remember the person you are taking care of and be sensitive and attentive to their individual and unique nursing needs. Provide humanistic care with genuine interest and compassion."

> *Nursing care is a science as well as an art. Therefore, the humanistic aspect must be intentional and deliberate in planning care that also includes therapeutic touch and cultural sensitivity and cultural competence.*

Dr. Munoz also added that, "As a nurse leader, one needs to have a vision for the future, set goals that are realistic and attainable. Be open to all opportunities to learn and accept challenges as opportunities for growth and self-fulfillment. Pursue higher education and have an impact on the education and training of young nurses. Seek a nursing leader as a mentor and be open to guidance and directions."

I asked Dr. Munoz if she believes great leaders are born or made by the circumstances they face, and according to her, "We are all born with God-given attributes, gifts, and talents. We may have the gift of a charismatic personality, but the leadership potential needs to be cultivated and learned. So, leaders are not born necessarily."

As a mentor, she was asked what advice she can provide to a protégé or mentee to achieve and sustain a meaningful professional relationship with their mentor, and her response was, "The mentor–mentee relationship is special and very fulfilling. There must be a collaborative match; therefore, one cannot assign these roles. Trust and credibility must be present in this relationship. The mentee needs to be open and accepting of challenges that would fit his/her own professional and personal goals. There also must be congruent philosophical values and personal beliefs so that a synergy is established." Dr. Munoz also added that mentoring a doctoral student is very fulfilling, especially as they go through the dissertation process and eventually earn their doctoral degree. I am very proud to call Dr. Cora Munoz my mentor.

My Life Well Lived

This is my narrative—a journey for over 50 years in the nursing profession, my experiences, challenges, and accomplishments. I have been increasingly interested and passionate about how we can finally address and eliminate health disparities and inequities in this society. Being equal is not acceptable nor sufficient. EQUITY is the goal.

During the COVID-19 pandemic, I found myself again in

> *Being equal is not acceptable nor sufficient. EQUITY is the goal.*

New York City where my daughter lives and where I started to live 52 years ago. This seems to be the circle of life. Although I continue to do a lot of virtual trainings, fully online teaching, and volunteering, I am able to spend time with my grandchildren. My daughter needed help in the care of my two grandsons, Newton Abel and Maxwell Abel, whom I love so dearly, as much as I love my only granddaughter, Isabel Jean. So, I have temporarily moved to New York City during the pandemic. The heart of a grandmother is a heart full of joy. Every moment with them is pure bliss. I am grateful for my siblings, especially my twin sister. Love of a family is priceless. The love of God is manifested through our family and our love for each other. I thank God for this journey, for being with me all along the way from the Philippines to New York City to Ohio and all my travels in between, and for all the people that I have met on this journey. All praise and glory to God!

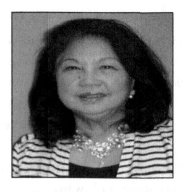

Cora Canlas-Munoz, PhD, RN

Dr. Cora Munoz is a professor emeritus and adjunct professor at Capital University. She is an author, academic scholar, consultant, national and international speaker, Fulbright scholar, diversity trainer, health advocate, and community worker. Her clinical specialty is psychiatric mental health and transcultural nursing with expertise in cultural competence, education and teaching nursing. She completed her master's in nursing education at Columbia University, Teachers College, in New York City with post-master's courses in psychiatric mental health nursing and her doctoral degree in counselor education with minor in nursing at the Ohio State University. She is currently the president of the Ohio Asian American Health Coalition. She has served for many years as the governor-appointed commissioner and served as vice-chair of the Ohio Commission on Minority Health. She is also a member of the Asian American Pacific Islander Advisory Council to the governor where she has served as chairperson of the health committee. In 2020, she was appointed by the governor to serve in the Minority Health COVID-19 Strikeforce and was the only Asian and the only RN represented in this Strikeforce Workgroup. She is currently the president of the Asian Festival Corporation and coordinated health screenings, health education, and community outreach for the Asian community. She was the founder of the Philippine Nurses Association of Indiana and the Philippine Nurses Association of Central Ohio in which she is a current board member in good standing. She has served as vice president for Culture of the Philippine American Society of Central Ohio and also served as board member of this organization. Dr. Munoz has received numerous accolades and awards as an outstanding nurse educator and community leader. She has received three Fulbright scholarships for the specialist program. She continues to teach transcultural nursing and provides trainings for cultural competency in health for various health disciplines. She was a nationally certified trainer for Chronic Disease Self-Management Program (CDSMP), a Stanford University evidence-based curriculum. Currently she is a certified trainer for culturally and linguistically appropriate services (CLAS) standards and the CARE curriculum through Multiethnic Advocates for Cultural Competency. She continues to be a nationally certified trainer for mental health first aid certified by the National Behavioral Health Council both in live, blended, and virtual curriculum. Dr. Munoz is currently an adjunct professor at Capital University and Mt. Carmel College of Nursing in Columbus, Ohio. She has been a nurse educator for over 40 years and a national trainer in areas of transcultural health, mental health, global health, psychiatric nursing and psychosocial issues, cultural competency, and diversity.

13

Equity in Nursing: Through the Eyes of an Immigrant

Karen Ofafa, MPH, BSN, RN, CSSBB, CPHQ

Why the Nursing Profession?

This was one of my favorite icebreaker questions while facilitating nurse leader workshops. Yet I had never personally fully reflected on my journey until the editors of this book invited me to share my story. Given the impact of COVID-19 on the frontline nursing workforce, and the obvious fact that I am not on the frontlines, I felt unworthy of this opportunity. However, upon reflection, I realized that the pandemic has left the bedside nurses hopeless and burnt out. I thought it was worthy for these nurses to know what the rest of us are doing to support them, that sharing my journey might give a nurse being pushed into early retirement a different nursing perspective to consider. I hope that after reading this chapter, you realize that there are opportunities beyond the bedside if you choose to consider them. I also hope that together, we can continue to push for equity in nursing. Lastly, I hope that any international student considering a career in health care can gain some insight from my journey! Editors, you are appreciated!

Jomo Kenyatta International Airport, February 1999

We simply do not know what the future holds.
—Peter L. Bernstein

I thought this day would never come. I had been counting down days for a while now. But when the day got here, I wanted to bail. In a few hours, I would be boarding an international flight for the first time. I was leaving my family and friends and going to start over in a place unfamiliar to me. I sat on the bed I shared with my sister Bertha. I was going to miss her dearly. Then, I heard my mom's voice calling me, "Nafula, it is time to go." Nafula is my middle name. It is common for parents to use middle names back home.

Traveling abroad was a big deal back then. Everyone wanted to see me off. My parents had rented a bus, and several relatives provided their cars for the ride to the airport. Led by my dad, our little convoy headed for the airport. I felt a million butterflies in my stomach. After checking in with my parents, I returned to bid my family farewell. My parents then escorted me to my gate. I sobbed! At the gate, my mom prayed. Dad reminded me that my connection was in London, but my luggage would be delivered to my destination. We hugged for a very long time, and I was off to chase the American dream.

Nairobi, Kenya, 1978–1999

I was born and raised in Nairobi, the capital city of Kenya. My parents Angela Ashihundu and Zakayo Paul Ashihundu were both born and raised in the western part of Kenya usually referred to as the village. My parents met and got married in Nairobi, then moved from the village to Nairobi in the 70s to look for better opportunities. Everyone from their generation dreamt of leaving the village life and getting a good job in Nairobi. My parents, being the pioneers in their families to accomplish this goal, provided needed support for their families. The younger generation supporting the older generation is a cultural norm back in Kenya.

My parents had five children: Bertha and Bernard (twins), Eric, me, and my youngest brother Emmanuel. Except Emmanuel, all of us went to boarding schools when we got to middle school. School was in session for 3 months, and we got a month break for holidays. Back in Kenya, boarding school was a popular and ideal option. For me, it was okay. I enjoyed all the back-to-school shopping, receiving pocket money, and visiting days (when parents would visit with their children). Boarding school made me very independent at a very early age. This setting was beneficial for parents because it provided students with an educational environment, opportunity to learn independence, availability of educational resources, and a curriculum that encompassed sports. For parents, this format allowed them to be able to navigate parenting and working concurrently. As a family, we had a very close relationship. I'm not sure if this is attributed to the time apart, but it was perfect.

Life was great as a kid. If my parents hustled, I never noticed it, but I know that they did. They were the kind of people that were generous, content, positive, God-fearing, and hardworking. My siblings and I were lucky to have been raised in such an environment. My parents both worked full time, and my dad ran a business on the side. With time, my parents also built a home in the country with the hopes of leaving the city life and retiring. They consistently shared that their desire was to support us until high school and then retire. It is normal in our culture for people to have a home in the city and a retirement home in the country. My parents were also well versed with educational opportunities abroad and encouraged us to excel in our studies so that we could qualify for educational opportunities in the United States.

University Education in Kenya: The Reality

I have two children: Katelyn (9) and Isaiah (13). What Katelyn wants to do when she grows up varies by the day. I was the same way, at least until school. I went from flight attendant to accountant and then to a chemistry teacher because my teachers had me tutoring chemistry to other students. I knew that a decision was necessary prior to college. However, the reality was that the Kenyan educational system at that time had major limitations. In fact, enrolling at a university of your choice for a program you desired was a rare occurrence. Kenya lacked this kind of academic freedom back in the late 90s. We had one university in 1960 and only five public universities in 2005 (Clark, 2015).

At some point in high school, I made the realization that I loved and excelled in natural sciences. I realized that opting for a career in the medical field would be rewarding. With support from my parents, we applied for some universities and decided to go with one in the same state as my brother Eric. Eric had left for the United States prior and was in Nebraska. I would be joining Eric at Bellevue University as a biology major with premedicine as my focus.

The American Dream

The 8-hour flight from Nairobi to London was uneventful. In London, I found my gate and boarded my connecting flight. I anticipated that I would experience some culture shock, but it came sooner than I expected. As I walked down the aisle, I felt the stares. Everyone wanted to start a conversation about my braided hair and others asked if they could touch it. "You have an accent"—this was the first of the many times I will hear this phrase. I was nervous. I fell asleep on the flight. The next time I opened my eyes, we were landing. The ground was white. I had read about snow but never seen it. I was exhausted. I made my way to the gate and saw Eric and his friends waiting for me. I was excited for the reunion. We hugged and Eric gave me a jacket. It was heavier than any jacket I had owned. It was very cold outside!

There was a significant amount of culture shock for the first few months. The food was different and abundant. I didn't starve growing up, but food was available when we needed it. We drank milk and water and saved soda and juices for special occasions, but in America, people could have these drinks with every meal. Growing up, we had one family car, a house phone, and only my parents had cellphones. Here, most houses had multiple cars in the driveways, and everyone had a cellphone. I had been washing my own clothes since I was in fifth grade, and my siblings and I took turns to do chores. I encountered kids who didn't do chores or, if they did, they got an allowance. Most houses had machines to wash clothes, dishes, or boil water. There was a drive-through for everything: the bank, the restaurant, and sometimes even the mailbox. I also had to adapt to American grammar, vocabulary, and pronunciation since my base was British English. Having a brother pave the way was a blessing.

Bellevue University, 1999–2003

My college classes eventually started, and I was enjoying them. Eric had a lineup of friends who would ensure I got to where I needed when he wasn't available. I also networked and focused on becoming independent. Eventually, I learned how to drive on the right side of the road. I was also making necessary adjustments and assimilating. I was an international student already paying exorbitant fees and needed to start supporting myself financially, so I applied for a student work permit and worked hard during my spare time.

During my junior year, I began to research my next steps for medical school application. I quickly learned that applying to medical school on an international student visa was not a favorable option. If accepted, I would either need to secure funding privately or show proof of funds to cover my education (Association of American Medical Colleges, n.d.). Yet, if I did not get into medical school in time, I would risk being in violation of my immigration status. The United States Citizenship and Immigration Services (USCIS) requires that a student on a visa be enrolled as a full-time student (USCIS, 2020). UCSIS grants students options to work during and between degree programs. Unless I acquired U.S. residency or citizenship, I would need to explore a different career path. I scratched medical school as an option. I could always revisit this.

The Art of Nursing

> *Be who God meant you to be, and you will set the*
> *world on fire.*
>
> —St. Catherine of Siena

I was awarded a bachelor of science in biology in the fall of 2003. I had applied for optional practical training (OPT), an authorization provided by USCIS that allows international students to work in an area directly related to their degree. Upon receiving OPT, I was hired as a hematology technician at a private chemistry laboratory in Nebraska. I finally had a real job, making the most I had ever made. However, working in the laboratory full time was not where my passion was. I did not feel like I belonged there. I needed to spend some time at the hospital learning about other existing opportunities. Sometime in 2003, I decided to pursue phlebotomy certification and use the opportunity to shadow other healthcare professionals. I also made this goal clear to my manager, who was able to accommodate my request. During my time as a phlebotomist, I found that I had more encounters with nurses than physicians in the patient care areas. The nurse-to-patient bond was obvious and lit a fire in me. It was obvious that nurses were the leaders at the bedside. This fueled my passion. I fell in love with the art of nursing.

Nursing Program Admission, 2004

I am not sure exactly when nursing accelerated programs came into existence, but 2004 was the first I heard of them. To be considered for a nursing accelerated program, you had to have a bachelor's degree and have met all the nursing prerequisites. These programs were all baccalaureate or higher and offered only core nursing courses. The courses themselves were accelerated. Most of them ran approximately 12 to 18 months for the entire program, and not every state had one. At this time, I had met my now husband, Waka Ofafa, and we were considering an out-of-state move. Together, we looked through a few programs and luckily, with a biology degree, I did not need any prerequisites for most programs. Our goal was to find a program with a fall 2004 admission date and one I could complete with no student loans. We applied and after going through acceptance letters, we decided to go with Grand Canyon University (GCU) in Arizona. It was a perfect fit. That year, we moved from Nebraska to Arizona, and in August 2004, I started the program. Our cohort was the first nursing accelerated program for GCU. I was in for an adventure.

Grand Canyon University, August 2004–February 2006

I cannot compare the time in nursing school to any time I had already spent in college; it was unique. Our cohort started with about 26 students and ended with 22. The time commitment was a huge barrier to most, especially those who had children or other family needs. School was full time, and clinicals happened during the week or weekends. Being unemployed was an admission prerequisite. Most figured out a way around this.

There was a lot of diversity in our class. Most students were second degree students. A lot of us had healthcare backgrounds. Some, like me, had done some type of patient care. We also had others with no healthcare experience. Our very first class was gerontology. It was everything about taking care of the elderly. We would learn the concepts and then demonstrate. The transformation for those who did not have healthcare experience was remarkable. It was fun to observe.

We had some amazing and experienced instructors who provided a wealth of knowledge and seemed to understand where we were coming from. One professor really stood out; she was a student favorite. Out of the concurrent classes we took in each block, she taught at least one. This professor was knowledgeable, personable, and empathetic. If a student did not have a babysitter and needed to bring her kid to class, she would adapt and incorporate that kid into the pediatric component and make the kid feel useful. She also helped us sift between what we needed to know to pass the nursing boards versus the knowledge we needed to be safe and competent clinicians. Our class came with brilliant students, but there was a lot of information to cover in a very short timeframe. I remember during our pharmacy course some students had C grades, and it led to a state of panic. This professor came to their rescue, uttering, "C means continue in nursing school. So put that grade behind you and focus on what you need to work on." She did not teach us to get As, but she taught us to grasp concepts. When it came to the higher level, more specialized courses, students questioned why that depth of knowledge was necessary for an area they would not specialize in. This professor would remind us, "This program is accelerated, not abbreviated. So go ahead and open your books, and let us continue." She made nursing school tolerable and fun! She was the reason we made it!

A lot happened in these 18 months. I planned my wedding, some students got married, some had grandchildren, and some had their children move away to college. But we celebrated all these things together. We were family! The summer during nursing school, I got some dreadful news from Kenya. My older brother Bernard had passed away in a car accident. I was devastated. Funerals in my culture could be a month-long celebration. The program did not allow any amount of time away, since most of our courses were 6 weeks long. Bereavement in America as I know it is usually 3 to 5 days. It would take me at least 2 days to get home and 2 days to get back. Going meant altering my course of study. I had to make the hardest choice I have ever had to make. I decided to miss my brother's funeral so that I could complete the program. But this isn't unique to me; other immigrants are constantly faced with having to make this choice. Healing took me a while, but I had the necessary support.

A Real Nurse (RN), 2006

> *I solemnly pledge myself before God and in the presence of this assembly, to pass my life in purity and to practice my profession faithfully. I will abstain from whatever is deleterious and mischievous, and will not take or knowingly administer any harmful drug. I will do all in my power to maintain and elevate the standard of my profession, and will hold in confidence all personal matters committed to my keeping and all family affairs coming to my knowledge in the practice of my calling. With loyalty will I endeavor to aid the physician in his work, and devote myself to the welfare of those committed to my care.*
>
> —The Florence Nightingale Pledge
> (Gretter, 1893)

In February of 2006, we completed our journey! I felt content. I was proud of my accomplishment. It was time to prepare for the boards.

I had enjoyed clinical rotations in nursing school. We had specific objectives, but I also took the time to observe the flow in the units, the patient's acuity, the cohesion on the nursing unit, nurse and patient attitudes, accessible resources, and the skill mix on the unit. To me, this was an opportunity to get a feel of the world I was going to be joining. I enjoyed my time in the critical care settings. I loved the fast pace, ambiguity, and complex care. After my nursing school graduation, I put in a few applications for new graduate registered nursing positions and specifically looked for organizations that would sponsor me to become a U.S. resident. This was critical. I had 12 months to either use an OPT or enroll in a more advanced degree, which I did not plan to do. I was shocked to get offers from two emergency departments (ED) immediately. One was a trauma hospital, and they were going to sponsor me to become a U.S. resident. Right there, I took a breath. Only a student on a visa can understand the burden lifted when one is offered residency or citizenship. These job offers came before I sat for my boards and gave me the pressure I needed. I passed my boards in April of 2006, 2 months after graduation.

John C. Lincoln ED: Trauma 1

I started working for John C. Lincoln Trauma Hospital in their ED that month. Transitioning from academia to practice was a learning curve, but I embraced it. It was a hard first year. I learned that I cannot save every patient and that every patient we lost was not my fault. I learned that there are more drownings in Arizona than I ever thought of, and I took this pain home with me every day. I was shocked by how many shootings we have in America, where I thought it was very safe. Yet not every day was hard. We saved a lot of patients. I recall a kid who came in complaining of buzzing in his ear. When we shined a light, there was a live insect in full motion in his ear. We took it out alive. He was a brave kid. We caught a lot of strokes early. We saved near-drowning kids. We taught parents of newborn children what an emergency was. There was a lot of good! I learned that as a nurse you cannot

> *I learned that as a nurse you cannot make assumptions, and you need to be aware of your unconscious bias.*

make assumptions, and you need to be aware of your unconscious bias. The lives we saved kept me sane!

Waka and I had some big changes a few years later. We bought our first home, he started nursing school, and we had Isaiah. I also switched hospitals with the move but remained in the ED setting. During my time in ED, I functioned in the capacity of an ED nurse, trauma nurse, and team lead. I also had the opportunity to work as a registry nurse and travel from hospital to hospital working both ED and telemetry to get that experience. During my ED tenure, I also received a few certifications including the Trauma Nurse Core Course (TNCC) certification. This work brought me enjoyment, but I wanted to continue exploring. With a background in biology and nursing, public health seemed like the next natural step for me to take. I decided to pursue a master's degree in public health.

Nursing Beyond the Bedside: Blood Systems Inc., 2009–2013

One of the most favorable things about nursing is the wide range of opportunities it offers. Upon graduation with a master's in public health in 2009 from Walden University, I transitioned from my full-time RN position to a position at Blood Systems (a blood bank) as a medical affairs counselor. My role was to counsel blood donors whose blood tested positive for transfusion-transmitted diseases. I was also involved in other processes that included donor eligibility criteria and donor deferral, and we served as the hotline for donation centers if they needed an emergency nurse to address donor reactions. Part of our role was also to report positive results to the state. The donor testing focused on Human Immunodeficiency Virus (HIV), hepatitis, syphilis, West Nile virus, dengue, Chagas disease, and malaria.

After a couple years of shadowing our blood bank physicians, I got involved with data analysis and trending. Specifically, my interest was on malaria. I grew up with this disease and thought I understood the pathology. Back home, malaria was common and treatable. People would be considered free from disease in a few weeks. I was curious why someone would test positive for malaria with no recent documentation of travel to a malaria-infected country. I explored this donor data and identified that most of these donors recorded that they were born in or had lived in the countries with malaria. With the help of my medical directors, I put together a study. As part of the study, we found that they all reported having malaria at some point, and one had it 40 years prior. I put together an abstract and submitted it to the American Association of Blood Banks (AABB). It was accepted, and I was invited for an oral presentation. Following that, my role and responsibilities were shifted, and I worked directly with the medical directors analyzing infectious disease trends, doing data analysis, managing multiple projects, and managing staff. This was also an opportunity for me to enhance my analytical skills, so I decided to pursue a certification in statistics. At that time, in addition to working full time at the blood bank and pursing a certification, I was practicing 24 hours a month as a nurse in the ED to keep up my clinical skills. This became a bit of a challenge to navigate when our daughter, Katelyn, was born in 2012. I stopped working at the ED for good.

In 2013, I graduated from my statistics program and received a Six Sigma Black Belt Certification from Arizona State University. At that point, I had been at the blood bank for 5 years and gained a lot. I had authored and coauthored a few abstracts and two manuscripts in the Journal of Blood Banking. I had gained new knowledge regarding transfusion diseases that I did not have prior. Since blood banking is highly regulated, I developed an interest in quality, regulatory processes, and outcomes. My career was just getting started.

To Err is Human

The National Academy of Medicine (previously called the Institute of Medicine) released their groundbreaking reports *To Err is Human* (1999) and *Crossing the Quality Chasm* (2001) before I was a nurse, but I was very familiar with these reports. As a registry nurse traveling to different hospitals, I had experienced some of the issues documented in these reports. I didn't know how I could impact these issues as a bedside nurse, but it was always at the back of my mind. The training I had received for the Black Belt Certification gave me more insight into current quality issues and how these could be addressed.

By the time I left Blood Systems, healthcare organizations had experienced some significant transformations since my time at the bedside. Some were adapting Lean and Six Sigma principles. Others were aiming to be high reliability organizations (HROs). Quality care and patient safety were at everyone's forefront. I needed to be part of this movement.

Versant Competency Solutions, 2014–2018

I found Versant Competency Solutions in 2014. When the president of Versant shared their mission and how they operationalize it, I immediately felt a sense of belonging. I knew that if I wanted to advocate for patient safety and quality care, this is where I needed to be. I was hired as a performance and outcomes consultant. My job was to partner with healthcare organizations and help them improve their health outcomes. This included transitioning new nurses from academia to the clinical setting, transitioning nurses from one unit to a higher acuity unit, enhancing the organization's nursing recruitment and increasing their retention, decreasing their turnover, and improving their patient safety. Additionally, we also supported leadership and preceptor development through the workshops we facilitated. I would collaborate with the leadership team (C-Suite) at an organization to complete a needs assessment, then, depending on the results, provide the needed support. Each organization was unique, and the programs were adapted to meet their needs. I traveled to various hospitals sometimes weekly to implement programs, conduct focus groups, round on patient care units, and review the organization's outcomes with the hospital executive team and nurse leaders.

I realized that nursing looks very different when you are outside looking in. Visiting different hospitals of different capacities gave me great insight. I learned that nurses are passionate about their jobs, but some sometimes lack the resources to demonstrate that. Nurses intend to provide safe patient care, but sometimes they are stretched too thin and sometimes have an error in judgment. Nurses are taught to advocate for their patients but then get frowned upon when they advocate for themselves. I also made some positive discoveries. Leaders want to reward and recognize nurses but sometimes must get creative with the rewards. If leaders understand nursing issues, they will provide the needed support. The states with mandated nursing staffing ratios have different problems from other states. I also realized that more parties are needed at the table to address these issues.

Embracing Adversity

*Nothing is impossible, the word itself says
"I'm possible."*

—Audrey Hepburn

Growth happens when we are challenged. For me, my challenges have become my defining moments. As a minority on a student visa, I was unable to commit to the medical school application process. Consequently, I did not become a physician. However, this adversity put me on the nursing path. I have been able to do more, be more, and give more as a nurse. I have also continued to grow and believe I still have potential.

Upon moving to the United States, I assimilated quickly. However, I had to give up my cultural views and cultural values and had to adapt to doing things a different way. My behaviors are now defined by the U.S. norms and not necessarily my cultural norms. Despite how challenging this might have been, it has been the best cultural training I will ever receive. As a nurse, it has made me more culturally sensitive and more aware of others cultural needs. I have been able to empathize with patients from a different culture. I appreciate their cultural views and incorporate them into care when and if they do not negatively impact their care.

> *Growth happens when we are challenged.*

Another challenge I routinely experience has to do with the diversity in my professional experience. Each role I have had is unique, but I see the alignment between the roles. Not every hiring team might see that. Sometimes I am told I am too clinical for a role, or that it appears that I would thrive more as a data analyst, or maybe I need more bedside experience. However, this has not been a barrier for me. I have been able to find opportunities when I needed to. I think it usually comes down to being able to articulate what skills I have and what I am looking for in a role.

Financing my education was also a bit of a challenge. My parents could have financed it if it came down to it. But I chose to support myself so they could take care of other priorities. School is much easier if you are not chasing a job, but that is what I needed to do. I made many compromises back then that have paid off greatly.

A Journey of Opportunities

Opportunity is missed by most people because it is dressed in overalls and looks like work.
—Thomas Edison

My diverse background has been my greatest opportunity. My skillset is unique, and that has frequently put me in a position of having a choice among job offers. For me, diversity has been an opportunity for me to stand out. I have also been exposed to influential people who have impacted my professional journey.

> *My diverse background has been my greatest opportunity.*

It is unusual for a new graduate nurse to start their first career in a critical or high acuity unit, but I was offered the opportunity and sponsored to be a U.S. resident. Not many organizations sponsor nonresidents, and not all professions qualify to be able to sponsor. This was an opportunity of a lifetime, and I eventually became a U.S. citizen in 2011.

I have also had the opportunity to be an accreditation appraiser for the American Nurses Credentialing Center's Practice Transition Accreditation Program (PTAP) and, as part of a team, reviewed evidence of organizations' work when they applied for PTAP accreditation. I have also been asked to review different processes outside my regular job at different points of my career and recommend enhancements.

I have also had opportunities to educate, mentor, and coach. Right after nursing school, I supported a small college, teaching the practical portion of the certified nursing assistant course. Additionally, while working for Blood Systems, they sponsored me together with a few medical directors to travel to Kenya and teach novice researchers how to conduct research. This was a weeklong course, and by the time we left, everyone had identified a study topic and data set and written an abstract. It was fulfilling. These relationships have given me more than I have given my mentees. I would not have had this exposure if I had not become a nurse.

Lastly, I had an opportunity to visit my congresswoman in Washington, DC, and bring up healthcare issues. During that visit, I focused on funding for nursing programs and healthcare documentation updates to allow nurses and providers more time with patients.

Milestones

> *We are what we repeatedly do. Excellence, then, is not an act, but a habit.*
>
> —Will Durant

My biggest accomplishment has been my contribution to the nursing profession. I have found pleasure in serving, leading, and advocating for others, but giving back to the profession has been the most fulfilling. I have given back by contributing to the body of knowledge through research; I have served as an educator, a mentor, and most recently, as a volunteer giving COVID-19 vaccinations in The Bahamas.

I have also grown as a professional. Ten years ago, I would never have imagined having a conversation with a chief executive officer about how an organization can do better or speaking with a provider about what they need to do to improve their patient compliance. I have learned that we are a team and working for the same goal. If I have something to bring to the table, it is appropriate to speak with my superiors. I continue to try and find the balance between parenting, working full time, school, and giving back!

Current Role: Cigna

Sometime in 2019, I left Versant. I had been on the road a lot. Isaiah and Katelyn were doing more activities, and Waka was single-handedly holding the fort down while working 12-hour shifts as an ICU nurse.

I joined Cigna in 2019 as a quality analyst specifically leading the Arizona market. On a day-to-day basis I ensure, together with our Accountable Care Organization (ACO) partners, that customers are receiving the highest quality care from our providers. The quality team at Cigna is responsible for accreditation, health plan performance and clinical initiatives implementation. Collectively, we ensure that we maintain or improve our accreditation scores, customers receive quality care, our health plan ratings remain competitive, and we implement clinical initiatives wherever appropriate to improve member compliance. The market leads analyze and trend the health plan data annually to identify any patterns. We then share findings with our medical executives and together collaborate with our ACOs on what is needed to improve health outcomes.

Doctor of Education, 2021–2023

I am currently pursuing a doctoral degree at Aspen University. I started considering a terminal degree a few years ago while consulting. While I have leadership experience from on-the-job training, I knew there was more to learn that can only be gained with a more formalized education. My goal is to graduate as a doctor of education (EdD) in healthcare administration with an emphasis on organizational development. There are two main doctoral tracks, and one of them is a doctorate in philosophy (PhD), which focuses on research and educational theories. I wanted to focus on education in professional practice, which is what the second track, EdD, focuses on.

Career Challenges

One of my biggest challenges has been having to decline opportunities that would advance my career but do not require a nursing license. When I market myself, I am first a nurse then a professional competent in analysis, public health, research, and Six Sigma methodologies. One can work in public health and be a Six Sigma Black Belt project manager, an analyst, or even a researcher in a healthcare organization without needing to be a licensed nurse, especially if the job responsibilities are not directly related to nursing. Some of these non-nursing positions came with significant compensation. However, my state board of nursing requires a nurse to practice nursing or complete a refresher course to maintain their license. I am not willing to give up my license for career advancement at this time.

Even though this is the norm, navigating parenting while working full time has been one of the challenges I have learned to manage. While I am not required to clock in and out and haven't been for a long time, I do often have time-sensitive deliverables. Spring is our busy season in my current role, and sometimes I can end up working 10-hour days at that time. I am learning to step away if I need to and not bring work to family engagements. It is a balance!

As a leader, I have often been challenged with managing up or managing my leaders' expectations. I think the issue here has do with my cultural background. I grew up with the mentality that your superiors (parents, leaders, older relatives) were always right, and your opinions might be taken as you trying to challenge them. I love coming up with more efficient ways to manage processes. I have had to constantly remind myself that I am the one doing the work, and I need to be able to articulate how to get it done more efficiently. Luckily, I have never been on a team or under a leader that does not want feedback.

In fact, one of my leaders used to say, "If you can't add to what I know or tell me how to do it better, why should I hire you?" I think nurses should allow themselves permission to speak up.

> *My mentality on the job has always been, "Show me where you want to go, and I will figure out how to get you there."*

My mentality on the job has always been, "Show me where you want to go, and I will figure out how to get you there." I take initiative on projects and function best when I am allowed to be creative with getting that work done. For the most part, this mentality is allowed. But often we tend to provide spreadsheets, templates, and line-by-line guides and not allow nurses to think outside the box. This becomes a challenge when there is advancement, especially with technology, and employees find ways to create work-arounds. We need to promote critical thinking and not be afraid to use technology to our advantage.

Opportunities for Nurses

While 2020 was designated as the year of the nurse (World Health Organization, 2020) and nurses continue to be called heroes, very little has been done to improve their motivation to work and their confidence in the profession. Nurses are often described as caring, flexible, adaptable, empathetic, resilient, confident, and understanding and dubbed advocate, coordinator, and communicator, to name a few. However, these qualities have been put to the test with the emergence of the COVID-19 pandemic. COVID-19 continues to impact the future of nursing and specifically the future of the bedside nurse. As mentioned

> *Our government needs to be a part of the solution to healthcare issues.*

earlier, nurses are losing momentum, and some are being forced into early retirement. It is time we as nurse leaders articulate the challenges our bedside nurses are facing.

Another opportunity we have as leaders is being able to bring up our nursing issues to Congress or to our elected representatives. This may require persistence and strength in numbers, but it is an appropriate platform and the only way for our voices to be heard by people who can impact change. Our government needs to be a part of the solution to healthcare issues.

Nursing has a lot of opportunities, but I am not sure we have done a great job educating nurses about them. A lot of bedside nurses might not be aware that they can be part of hospital committees, their shared governance, or that the hospital has forums where they can share their concerns and best practices. Additionally, some nurses are not aware that there are opportunities outside the hospital. Nurses can join academia, consulting firms, the state, insurance companies, and other private organizations. Nonmedical industries are now hiring their own medical concierge team or nurses for nursing-related tasks.

While I recommend nurses advance their education, I think the industry has an opportunity to better educate nurses on meaningful educational advancements. In my opinion, all nurses need a bachelor's degree. Associate nursing degrees do not usually encompass the leadership competencies taught in a bachelor's program. Beyond that, I would focus on where that training might take you. Certifications in areas of your specialty might be more useful if you are not planning to apply that degree or advance in your role beyond the bedside. Health care is continuously evolving. Standards and practices are continuously changing. It is best to gain new knowledge when it is most applicable.

Recommendations for Equity in the Future

You can't lead without influence, and you can't have influence if you're not a leader.
—Unknown

During my consulting tenure, what I heard frequently from nurses was that they were sharing issues over and over with no resolution. Nurses at the bedside sometimes have power without authority or are expected to influence but aren't allowed to lead. To increase opportunities for nurses, I recommend that we review the following areas.

Just Culture

Quality issues and their impact on nurses has been well documented. The groundbreaking reports from the National Academy of Medicine (Institute of Medicine, 1999, 2001) opened our eyes to system failures that lead to quality-of-care issues. Sometimes, at the end of that system failure is a nurse who gets blamed for the issue. As industry leaders, we need to come together and address these quality issues at our organizations. Leaders need to promote a culture of safety. My recommendation is to standardize error reporting and ensure it is championed as nonpunitive.

Transitioning Nurses From Academia to Practice

There are significant inconsistencies in how nurses are transitioned into the profession. Nurses, just like physicians, come out of nursing school with a lot of generalized knowledge. The clinical experience required is also not standardized across the country, and not everyone gets the opportunity to experience all the basics you would expect to see within the first year. However, when they are hired on a unit, most often, the training is not customized to the individual. This leads to nurses being unable to demonstrate competence when left to care for a patient independently, subsequently compromising patient safety. When doctors or pharmacists complete their education, they spend some time in residency programs and demonstrate competence prior to becoming independent practitioners. This should be the same expectation for nurses. As leaders, we need to address the transition to nursing practice programs. My recommendation is that they are formalized and standardized across the country.

Diversity in the Nursing Workforce

According to Western Governors University (2019), there is a lack of diversity in the nursing workforce and minority groups represent only 20% of the workforce. From a 2017 survey conducted by the National Council of State Boards of Nursing, 80% of the nursing workforce is White/Caucasian, and 19.2% is any other ethnicity or race (American Association of Colleges of Nursing, 2019). This is seemingly an issue as our population continues to be diverse and needs a diverse nursing workforce to be able to address their issues. The American Association of Colleges of Nursing (2019) reinforces this by stating that culturally competent care is tied to a culturally diverse workforce. Patients feel connected and form relationships with caregivers of the same race, and this may lead to improved health outcomes. My recommendation is that we work on recruiting from our minority groups to ensure that the nursing workforce is representative of our diverse population.

Advancement Opportunities in Nursing

One thing nurse leaders and administrators need to be aware of is the importance of the role of the bedside nurse. The voice of the bedside nurse is what gets patients the care they need. Because of these bedside nurses, the patient's preferences are incorporated into their care; because of these nurses, the patient's family is involved in the patient's care; because of these nurses, the interprofessional team knows their role in this patient's care. We cannot lose sight of this.

Most nurses join the profession to care and advocate for their patients. These nurses are the leaders at the bedside. But what I saw while I was a consultant is that a good number of nurses lack the confidence to carry themselves around as leaders. We need to do a better job making these nurses feel like leaders.

What I recommend is that organizations make leadership opportunities and career advancement for these nurses more visible to them. The bedside nurse may have a calling to stay at the bedside. If that is the case, we need to involve them in leadership rounds, shared governance, or hospital committees and ensure that their needs and the needs of the patients they care for are being met. We need to include bedside nurse representatives in forums where decisions are made. The nurses at the bedside are operationalizing the hospital's mission. The leadership team creates a plan, and the bedside nurses and others at the front lines execute that plan. Nurses need a seat at the table!

> **Nurses need a seat at the table!**

***

To my husband, Waka, and our children, Isaiah, and Katelyn,
Waka, may we continue to explore the world together! Katelyn and Isaiah, we are so proud of who you are becoming! This is just the beginning. Love you all to the moon and back!

To my parents, Zakayo and Angela Ashihundu,
Thank you for teaching me how to love, give, and work hard. I am everything I am because of you guys! I love you both dearly!

To my siblings, Bertha, Bernard, Eric, and Emmanuel,
Bernard, you are missed greatly. Bertha, Eric, and Emmanuel, I have everything because I have you guys! Love you!

To my fellow nurses, the ones who keep daring greatly, please always remember . . .

> It is not the critic who counts: not the man who points out how the strong man stumbles or where the doer of deeds could have done them better. The credit belongs to the man who is actually in the arena, whose face is marred by dust and sweat and blood, who strives valiantly, who errs, who comes short again and again, because there is no effort without error and shortcoming; but who does actually strive to do the deeds; who knows the great enthusiasms, the great devotions, who spends himself in a worthy cause; who at the best, knows, in the end, the triumph of high achievement, and who, at the worst, if he fails, at least fails while daring greatly . . .

—Theodore Roosevelt

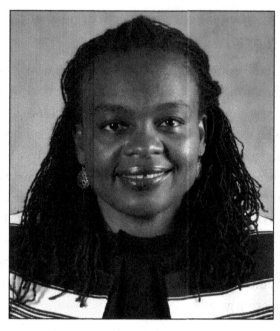

Karen Ofafa, MPH, BSN, RN, CSSBB, CPHQ

Karen Ofafa, MPH, BSN, RN, CSSBB, CPHQ, is a quality analyst at Cigna responsible for providing oversight and leading efforts to improve health plan outcomes for the Arizona market. Her previous roles include emergency room nurse, transfusion medicine researcher, and most recently consultant for hospital executives in multiple hospitals to implement solutions to improve patient safety.

Karen has demonstrated success with improving nurse retention, implementing competency-based workforce solutions, and improving healthcare quality. Karen has also served as a hospital accreditation peer reviewer and has authored publications focused on transfusion medicine research.

Karen is certified in Healthcare Quality and holds a Six Sigma Black Belt. She is an advocate for diversity in the nursing workforce and empowering nurses to lead beyond the bedside. She is currently enrolled in a doctorate in education program with an emphasis on healthcare administration leadership as she strives to make an impact in the future of nursing!

14

Ka Waiwai Aloha o Ko'u Makuahine

(The Life Lessons, Memories, Compassion, and
Spiritual/Emotional Gifts of My Mother)

Mary Frances Mailelauli'i Oneha, PhD, RN, APRN, FAAN

I Come From a Place

On a warm summer day on the north shore of O'ahu, Hawai'i, my
brothers and cousins, as children, were riding their bikes around
the farm. My cousin, 8 years old, fell and scraped his hands and
knees. He was hurt, and through his tears, he asked my brothers
to "call Mary." My brothers responded, "What do you need Mary
for?" My cousin replied, "'Cause she's a nurse." At the time, I was
volunteering at a hospital as a candy striper.

I was born in Honolulu and spent most of my childhood and
teenage years growing up on a farm at Waile'e, O'ahu. My father
worked at the dairy caring for the cows, from milking them early in
the morning to feeding them in the late afternoon. As children, we
enjoyed going to work with him to help milk and feed the cows and
wash the concrete pavement of the dairy after each workday. We
also enjoyed riding our bikes, hiking into the mountains, building
forts with our neighbors, and going across the street to swim in the
ocean. As we had no television reception or other electronic devices

at the time, we were always anxious to get out of the house. My father would whistle for us when it was time to come home for dinner. It was a distinct whistle and, as we lived in a remote area, we knew the whistle was coming from my father, and it was time to go home.

My Mother's *Hā* (Breath, Life)

While we spent time with my father and friends, my mother worked as a registered nurse at the community hospital in the evenings or nights. My mother recalled as she rode in the ambulance to get to an emergency, that there were no addresses; they found a location by the number of telephone poles along the roadway. In a small community hospital, nurses were assigned to a variety of duties and did what was needed within the hospital. This was the only emergency room and ambulance serving the entire north side of the island of Oʻahu at that time.

My mother eventually moved on to work for the Hawaiʻi State Department of Health Hansen's Disease Program at Hale Mohalu Hospital located about 28 miles from our home. She usually worked during the day or evening shifts. She also had the opportunity to travel to Kalaupapa on the island of Molokaʻi to work with the staff at the hospital serving those with Hansen's disease. She enjoyed her time with the patients and staff at Kalaupapa. My mother shared a funny story about one of her trips to Kalaupapa. As she was making her arrangements to fly into Kalaupapa, one of the patients offered his truck for her to get from the airstrip to the hospital. My mother asked, "How will I get the keys to your truck?" The patient responded, "Mrs. Oneha, I going leave it in the truck." My mother was astonished and said, "You not scared somebody going take your truck?" The patient laughed, "Mrs. Oneha, where they going?" Kalaupapa is a peninsula on the island of Molokaʻi, and the only way in or out is by plane, boat, or a hike or mule ride down a steep cliff. Currently, it is a national historical park to preserve the experiences of people forcibly sent there and to educate visitors about Hansen's disease and the hard lessons learned about the isolation of a community.

There were many days when we did not see her after school, we would then see her the next morning. As I got older and started high school, there were many instances when I would ask my mother to review my written papers on a particular subject by leaving them out overnight on the dining table with a note for her to review, so I could see her comments the next morning before I went to school.

My sisters and I traveled 2 hours by bus, each way, to high school. My father would wake us early in the morning, preparing breakfast and lunch before getting us out the door to the bus stop at 5:00 a.m. We would also have to leave school early to make the last bus heading to our home.

When I was in high school, my father became seriously ill and required renal dialysis. He and my mother attended classes so they could dialyze him at home. Once I graduated from nursing school, I assisted my father with this process until my mother returned home from work.

In hindsight, I think my mother being a nurse had a great impact on me. I knew by the time I was a freshman in high school that I was going to be a nurse and that all of my studies were focused in that direction. In addition, I also knew I was going to be a pediatric nurse. My father supported my choice to become a nurse, but he was hesitant about my move to the continental United States. On the other hand, my mother discouraged me from pursuing nursing as a career. She was concerned that I was "too quiet" and felt that nursing required one to be much more assertive.

Ka hana a ka mākua, o ka hana no ia a keiki (What Parents Do, Children Will Do)

—'Ōlelo No'eau #1295 (Pukui, 1983)

I volunteered at a small community hospital as a candy striper, then worked as a nurse's aide at various hospitals. As I completed my pre-nursing classes, many in these classes, which were very diverse, were concerned about whether they would be accepted to the bachelor of science nursing program at the University of Hawai'i, and several had a backup plan if they were not accepted. I did not have a backup plan. I applied and was accepted. Going through nursing school required a lot of resources and support, particularly in getting through clinical rotations at various sites, as I stayed in on-campus housing and did not have a car. I would ride with classmates, take the bus, or have my father drop me off or pick me up from various clinical sites. I enjoyed most of my clinical rotations; pediatrics was my favorite, as children were so interactive and resilient. Psychiatry was my most challenging and took time for me to process and understand. My world revolved around going to school and studying; there was no time for anything else. I just wanted to pass my courses and graduate. With the support of my family and classmates, I graduated with a bachelor of science degree in nursing in 1981 from the University of Hawai'i.

It was common for nursing students to be encouraged by faculty to practice in acute care adult settings after graduation. This was the setting that new graduates were expected to start in. There was no mention of long-term care, community health nursing, or pediatrics. I was interested in pediatrics and wanted to work at a hospital for children in Hawai'i. It was the first year this hospital recruited new graduates. There were three from my class recruited to work at this hospital. Most of our classmates went to acute care hospital settings serving adults and a few practiced at outpatient clinics. Unfortunately, I was recruited before I learned the results of my state board exam. I did not pass and was moved to a nurse's aide position. I continued to work as a nurse's aide until I was able to retake the exam and passed. I then moved to a registered nurse position. I was the only registered nurse working the night shift with a licensed practical nurse and a nurse's aide. My learning curve was steep, and I am indebted to these nurses for their support, guidance, and expertise. My 2 years at this hospital prepared me for other nursing positions, but they did not prepare me for the cultural differences I would experience.

I ka nānā no a ʻike (By Observing, One Learns)

—ʻŌlelo Noʻeau #1186 (Pukui, 1983)

Over the next 8 years, and after my father passed, I worked at two different pediatric hospitals; in Ohio for about 1 year and then in Washington state for 7 years. I am grateful for the opportunities nursing presented, as I gained experience in acute and critical care as a staff nurse, charge nurse, line management nurse, nursery nurse, and neonatal intensive care nurse. Each of these states and hospital settings were different. I was acutely aware that I looked different. I was darker than most—being of Native Hawaiian, Chinese, Scottish, and English descent. I used different words when communicating, such as local pidgin (influenced by the various peoples of Japanese, Filipino, Chinese, Portuguese, etc. descent that came to work on the plantations in Hawaiʻi) or

Hawaiian words. I made different dishes at potlucks and ate food that most were unfamiliar with, such as poi (taro that has been pounded to a pudding-like consistency), raw fish, lomi salmon (cubes of salmon with tomatoes and onions), and laulau (pork, chicken, fish, and/or sweet potato wrapped in taro leaves and steamed). While living in Ohio and Washington state, I would call my mother to ask why the same food looked and tasted different, only to understand that different ingredients were used or omitted. My move to Ohio in 1984 took me on a cross-country journey by car from California to Ohio with a friend who was of Japanese and Italian descent. It was an eye-opening experience to not be served at certain restaurants due to the color of our skin or maybe the shape of our eyes.

As I moved from Akron, Ohio, to Seattle, Washington, I became comfortable working nights and chose to work permanent nights rather than rotating shifts. I was hired the same day I interviewed at Seattle Children's Hospital, as the supervisor expressed disbelief that I preferred to work the permanent night shift, from 11:00 p.m. to 7:00 a.m. Nursing again presented multiple opportunities to work with families from across the Northwest and with different age groups, from infants to adolescents. This profession allowed me to experience how families responded to their child's diagnosis and how they prepared for discharge.

After several years with Seattle Children's Hospital, I was interested in continuing my education and pursuing a master of nursing degree with a focus on parent–child nursing and community health nursing. As acute care nursing in a hospital ended at the time of discharge, I was interested in understanding and experiencing how families lived and coped at home in their communities. As with my first admission to nursing school, I expected that it would be challenging to be admitted to the University of Washington master of nursing program. Fortunately, I applied and was accepted. It is not lost on me that I was likely, though I am not sure, one of very few applicants from an underrepresented racial group. I appreciated the gentle push from faculty, our stimulating discussions, and progressive assignments. My practicum experience in public health nursing afforded me exposure to the community, though I came to realize this was very different than my experience growing up in my family and community in Hawaiʻi.

Moving home to Hawaiʻi became a goal after completion of my master of nursing degree at the University of Washington in 1991. Needless to say, this move was a culture shock after being away from Hawaiʻi for 8 years. There are multiple cultures represented in Hawaiʻi, all with their own customs, ways, languages, thought patterns, and food. There were also several now-historical moments related to Native Hawaiian well-being that I missed while living away from Hawaiʻi. It took some time to get readjusted as I started working for the State of Hawaiʻi Department of Health Public Health Nursing Branch, serving a community in central Oahu as a public health nurse. I was more commonly known and referred to as "Roberta's [my mother] daughter" than my own name. Soon after, an opportunity to work in a joint position as faculty at the University of Hawaiʻi School of Nursing and at a federally qualified health center (FQHC), Waianae Coast Comprehensive Health Center (WCCHC), arose. The opportunity involved a multi-professional group of professionals and students learning at their academic setting and their assigned health center. I served as the clinical nursing specialist (CNS) on the project. I also had a nurse practitioner counterpart. Practicing with other health professionals, including social work, medicine, and public health, was a great experience. However, working in a joint position felt like having two full-time jobs that were a long distance from each other.

After 5 years on this project, I made the decision to only work at the health center. This health center served a majority Native Hawaiians on the west side of the island of Oʻahu. I had found my fit and remained there for nearly 20 years before moving on to another FQHC, Waimānalo Health Center, also serving a majority Native Hawaiians.

Hoʻi hou i ka iwi kuamoʻo (Return to the Backbone)

—ʻŌlelo Noʻeau #1024 (Pukui, 1983)

It was through this experience at the WCCHC that my focus as a nurse evolved to improving the health status of Native Hawaiians through education, research, and practice. Three years after graduating with my master's degree, I was interested in going back to school for a doctoral degree. I did not have the desire to move back to the continental United States and was very attached to remaining in Hawaiʻi for as much time as possible so I could discover how to best serve Native Hawaiian communities. I pursued my PhD at the University of Colorado Health Sciences Center

Hoʻi hou i ka iwi kuamoʻo (Return to the Backbone)

School of Nursing summer program and completed my dissertation at WCCHC, exploring a sense of place and its relationship to health as perceived and experienced by Hawaiian participants living in Waiʼanae. My studies and the support of faculty in Colorado were critical in advancing my nursing knowledge and its application to communities. I think it was in this setting that I began to truly find my voice and share my opinions and experiences. This was encouraged, yet I was hesitant, as I perceived my opinions and experiences to be so different from others. I drew on my experiences in Hawaiʻi, from the community I was working with, and from my mother's call to be more assertive.

While my experiences at each FQHC exposed the worst of people "knowing what's best" for communities or perpetuating stereotypes, it also highlighted the best of a community's resiliency, the generations of families and cultural practices that have thrived in these communities, and the healthcare personnel who are committed to service. Similar to how I felt during my academic experiences in just wanting to know and feel that I—and all the experiences I bring, from my ancestors to the present day—am valued, respected, and appreciated, so too do other Native Hawaiians. The challenges existing and opportunities available today include, first, that Native Hawaiians are the Indigenous or first peoples of the ʻāina (land) of Hawaiʻi and should be the first peoples to provide ʻike (knowledge) to solutions of problems affecting them. Second, Native Hawaiians should consistently be disaggregated and counted as a unique racial group. Next, resources to support communities experiencing the greatest inequities with chronic diseases or social determinants (inadequate housing, food insecurity, lack of or inadequate education, etc.) should be received by or awarded to the community or as close to the community as possible. Finally, the COVID-19 pandemic exacerbated what we already knew about health inequities, with populations who were devastated and challenged to understand what to do with educational materials and announcements primarily in English, identify where to isolate their multigenerational households with low income, and trust the source (the federal government) of historical distress. The exacerbation of high positive COVID-19 cases, lack of opportunities for isolation/quarantine, and a lack of confidence in COVID-19 vaccines were a plea for all of us to support and respect each other in meeting the needs of communities through appropriate, culturally relevant, innovative, and sustainable ways.

E kaupē aku no I ka hoe a kō mai (Put Forward the Paddle and Draw it Back. Go on With the Task That Is Started and Finish It)

—'Ōlelo No'eau #319 (Pukui, 1983)

Nursing needs to move in parallel with this call for equity. Ensure that all voices, skin colors, and eye shapes are encouraged, represented, and respected in education, research, and practice. Require that appropriate community voices are included in research proposals and applications. Ensure that there is equitable representation in the pool of nursing applicants, and if not equitable, identify the supports needed or strategies to close gaps.

> *E kaupē aku no I ka hoe a kō mai (Put Forward the Paddle and Draw it Back. Go on With the Task That Is Started and Finish It)*

I am fortunate that I have the opportunity to not only share these messages and expectations but to work to ensure they are operationalized. My mother, Roberta Anne Maile-lauli'i Oneha, of Native Hawaiian, Scottish, and English descent, was a 1957 graduate of the St. Francis School of Nursing, where she received her nursing diploma and worked as a registered nurse for 36 years. Her daughter, Mary

Frances Mailelauliʻi Oneha, "went all the way," as my mother described my career to her friends. Although she discouraged me from going into nursing, she provided unending support, guidance, teachings, and patience to see me through to my PhD and a fellowship in the American Academy of Nursing. My mother passed on September 2, 2021. This is the legacy she left, and I will be eternally grateful.

Ensure that all voices, skin colors, and eye shapes are encouraged, represented, and respected in education, research, and practice.

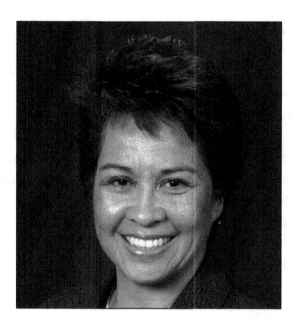

Mary Frances Mailelauliʻi Oneha, PhD, RN, APRN, FAAN

Mary Frances Mailelauliʻi Oneha has worked in community health centers for nearly 30 years and has served as the
chief executive officer of the Waimānalo Health Center since
2012. Her collaborative research and publication efforts with
other community-minded researchers have aligned with her commitment to improve the health of Native Hawaiians. Her most
recent community-based research project examined the added
value of Native Hawaiian healers and their healing practices integrated in primary care. She supports the perpetuation of Native
Hawaiian cultural practices in health care and advocates for
this value-added service in payment models. Dr. Oneha serves
on the Boards of the Na Limihana o Lonopuha Native Hawaiian
Health Consortium, AlohaCare, Hawaiʻi Primary Care Association,

and the Association of Asian Pacific Community Health Organizations. She received her PhD in nursing from the University of Colorado, a master of nursing from the University of Washington, and a bachelor of science from the University of Hawaiʻi. She is a 2018 fellow of the American Academy of Nursing, a 2016 inaugural inductee to the University of Hawaiʻi School of Nursing Hall of Fame, and a 2016 Hawaiian Civic Club of Honolulu Na Wahine Puuwai Aloha (women who give generously) honoree, and she was recognized by the White House in 2013 as an AAPI Woman Champion of Change.

15

Finding and Living My Passion

Shannon Whittington, MSN, RN, CCM

"I'm gonna be a nurse!" This was my declaration at the early age of five. Even when grown-ups would say to me, "Little girl, you'll change your mind when you grow up," my soul knew without a shadow of a doubt that this was my destiny. So, once I graduated from high school, I applied and was accepted into a nursing program. I must admit that obtaining my bachelor's degree in nursing was the hardest thing I've ever done. I remember sitting in class as a doe-eyed nursing student when the professor gave her welcome, or should I say warning, speech: "Look to your left, look to your right. Tomorrow that person probably won't be there." And sure enough, day after day, my class of 166 students would slowly dwindle to a mere 66. I somehow managed to hold onto my seat, though, through every obstacle, and trust me, there were many: insomnia, sleep deprivation, stress, acne, nausea, diarrhea, and the traumatizing mind games my professors would play, seemingly to set me up for failure. It seemed as if every hour not spent in class was spent studying for class or worrying that I was going to fail, be pulled into the professor's office for a verbal lashing, or experience public humiliation on the hospital floor. It was absolute misery day in and day out.

Each year, my university would organize a huge homecoming spectacular with parades, decorations, and lots of fun activities. Not that I had time to attend any of those things, but one day, I got a wild hair and decided to run for homecoming queen. I campaigned for several months, never once mentioning this to my professors for fear of their sabotage. My university had over 25 thousand students, so the chances of me winning were slim, but I figured why not give it a shot? And as luck would have it, one night on centerfield in front of the hugest crowd ever, they crowned me the winner. Getting my picture in the city paper made me somewhat of a local celebrity, and this popularity further fueled my professors' vision of me not being nurse material. After the crowning ceremony, a reporter called my house and asked me how I was planning to celebrate. I quickly replied, "I'm studying for an exam." And that's what I did. I never celebrated my homecoming queen victory.

Despite the many struggles, I kept trudging through until I eventually reached the final hurdle of passing boards. During those days, we had to drive to the state capital to take the test. It was 2 intense 8-hour days of pure torture. I remember stumbling out of the room feeling like my head was about to explode. And of course, everyone was asking me, "How did you do? Do you think you passed?" Honestly, I didn't think I passed. I have never been good at test taking, and I was certain that after 4 long years of studying, I was about to experience the biggest embarrassment and disappointment of my entire life. I would fulfill my professors' prophesies of ineptitude. Since the failure rate was so high, I was convinced I would be part of that statistic. I would sell shoes for the rest of my life.

I waited anxiously for months for my results. When I finally got the letter in the mail, my hands were shaking so much I didn't have the strength to stand, much less open the envelope. As I slowly slid my way to the floor, my mom ripped the envelope open and proudly announced, "Candidate passed!" I was in disbelief and utter shock. I was frozen. All that pain, studying, and personal sacrifice had finally paid off. In the end, it was all worth it, or so I thought.

After surviving the most brutal curriculum of my entire life, fear stalled my entry into practice. I began to unravel and seriously doubt myself and my ability to be a nurse. The negative tapes I heard during nursing school began to play on repeat in my head. "You aren't cut out to be a nurse, Shannon. Nursing isn't for you. Why don't you switch majors? You don't have what it takes to be a nurse." I was so fearful of setting foot on a hospital floor that I became the regional shoe sales leader at JCPenney! After all, if working as a nurse was as traumatic as nursing school, I wanted no part of it.

After 3 months, I finally garnered enough gumption to apply for a position at the local hospital. At the tender age of 22, I was taking care of very sick patients on a cardiology unit. I worked the 12-hour night shift for 7 days straight, and then I would be off for 7 days. Some of my coworkers weren't that welcoming—especially the older nurses who sneered at my bachelor's degree and local celebrity status. They accused me of becoming a nurse just so I could marry a doctor. Funny thing is, marrying a doctor had never crossed my mind. They scoffed at my limited clinical experience. I began to wonder, "Is this all there is? Further humiliation? Work, sleep, survive, repeat? Is this the destiny I dreamed of?"

Thankfully, I wasn't alone at my job. An LPN named Joyce took me under her wing and taught me everything I needed to know to keep up with the more tenured nurses: how to handle patients with psych issues, how to insert an NG tube, collect urine, administer nitroglycerin, and how to read EKG strips. More importantly, she taught me how to handle the nurses who weren't so nice. She taught me how to deal with bosses and bullying. I wouldn't have survived without Joyce.

At 24, I relocated to Atlanta and secured a position on a renal and hepatic transplant unit, but, yet again, it was not a pleasant experience. By this time, I had started a modeling career, and eventually, my coworkers started to see my picture in magazines and newspapers. I denied it by saying everyone has a twin, but that didn't last for long. This time around, I didn't have Joyce with me to make the days less brutal. But one day, something happened: My experience—and my gut—led me to a memorable milestone.

I was tending to a patient when I started to feel a sense of dread in the pit of my belly. Even though her vital signs were normal, something just didn't feel right. So I immediately cleared the room, and the next thing you know, just like that, my patient coded. Before this event, the other nurses never paid much attention to me. They thought I was on the slow side, being so country and all. What they didn't know was that I had spent 2 years as a cardiology nurse, and one thing I knew how to do, and do very well, was function during a code. I knew how not to panic, and I also knew how to anticipate the next med that would be pushed. I quickly started an IV on my crashing patient, got the drip going, got the crash cart, and put the board under her. Even though it had been a year since I was in a code, it came back to me like riding a bike. I saw two nurses staring at me from the corner of the room in disbelief. Thankfully, the patient survived. I earned a great deal of respect that day. Overnight, I was no longer the country bumpkin from Tennessee; I was now a knowledgeable and valuable member of the team.

Two years later, I moved to New York City and got a job on another cardiology unit. But even with the experience of working in one of the biggest cities and hospitals in the world, it still wasn't satisfying to me. I quit nursing three times. I even tried my hand at being a cater waiter, and I did that for 5 years. I eventually succumbed to the notion that I would never have career satisfaction as a nurse, and this was something I had to make peace with. As sad as this was for me, it was my grim reality for the next 20-plus years.

Something happened one day that would change this unpleasant reality, however, and I'm pretty sure being gay had a lot to do with it. On a random day like any other, my boss summoned me into her office and told me to "go check out some gender surgeries" at the local hospital and come back with a report. "I don't think it's gonna amount to much," she said. At the time, I had a boss you didn't say no to, so of course I said yes, never realizing that this yes would not only change the trajectory of my career but also my life. I proceeded to learn everything about gender-affirming surgeries for transgender patients. Before this, I didn't even know what those words meant! I immediately recognized my knowledge gap in this area, and after 20 long years of harboring trauma from nursing school, I gathered the courage to go back to school for my master's degree. My fear of failure was enormous, but I ended up graduating with a 4.0, and I will likely have my doctorate by the time you read this.

Over time, thankfully, I started to gain a feeling of satisfaction that never came close to being matched over the last 3-plus decades. Finally, I found my passion that I had craved for so many years, my passion to educate others on a topic that is sorely missing in our curriculums and practice. Did you know that in our curriculum, we, as nurses, average about 2 hours of training regarding LGBTQ+, if that? That's right: 2 measly hours to learn how to treat and care for members of such a large, unique, and diverse community.

As a nurse who is openly gay, I find this disturbing. It is vitally important to learn more about providing care for members of my community, particularly those who require gender-affirming surgeries and treatment. As a result, I have trained hundreds of nurses and clinicians on this topic, gained certifications, and have written and spoken about this all over the country as a consultant and author. I have developed a program from scratch for home care of the postoperative transgender patient. I eventually received numerous awards, city council funding, and over three million dollars for research. This experience has empowered me—and others—to provide the best possible care to the LGBTQ+ community.

I am finally in my sweet spot. Now, I spend my waking hours dreaming about changing how health care is delivered to my people. I dream of clinical transformation of nurses who can care for these patients without bias or discrimination. I know this is a tall order, much like winning homecoming queen, but maybe I might just win. I'm glad this passion has shown up at this later point in my career. It gives me hope that I can make a difference before I leave this world.

With nearly 10 million LGBTQ+ people in the United States alone, chances are we are working as healthcare providers as well as receiving care as patients right next to you.

With nearly 10 million LGBTQ+ people in the United States alone, chances are we are working as healthcare providers as well as receiving care as patients right next to you. I recommend that hiring managers consider hiring nurses who are from this community, and I also recommend internal stakeholders provide cultural competence training for their staff. In addition to fostering a true sense of equity for people of marginalized backgrounds, diverse teams have been proven to make better decisions, which means better outcomes for hospitals and patients. Despite the strides our society has made in the name of LGBTQ+ equity, there is still unaddressed disparity that needs attention.

As I look back over my career, from its highs to its lows, I realize that I have a tremendous vantage point and hope for the future of nursing. I know what it's like to be mistreated as a student and as a novice nurse. I know what it's like to be bullied, and I also know what it's like to be empowered to win. I know what it's like to contribute to this profession in a scholarly way. I'm confident that my fellow game changers and I can and will make a difference that will empower and educate the current and next generation of nurses and healthcare providers. Will you join me?

> *Fellow game changers and I can and will make a difference that will empower and educate the current and next generation of nurses and healthcare providers. Will you join me?*

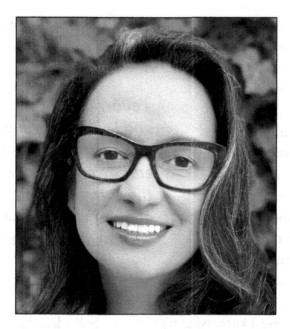

Shannon Whittington, MSN, RN, CCM

Shannon Whittington (she/her) is a speaker, bestselling author, consultant, and clinical nurse educator. Her area of expertise is LGBTQ+ person-centered care and LGBTQ+ workplace inclusion. Shannon has a passion for transgender health, where she educates clinicians in how to care for transgender individuals after undergoing gender-affirming surgeries. She received the Quality and Innovation Award from the Home Care Association of New York, Notable LGBTQ+ Leaders & Executives Award by Crain's New York Business, and International Association of Top Professionals Nurse of the Year Award. Shannon is a city and state lobbyist for transgender equality. You can follow Shannon on LinkedIn (https://www.linkedin.com/in/shannonwhittington/k) and

YouTube (ShannonWhittingtonConsulting). Upcoming book launches include *LGBTQ+: ABC's for Grown-Ups, Kindergarten for Nurses: 9 Essential Tips for Nurse Leaders,* and *Kindergarten for Leaders: 9 Essential Tips for Grown-Up Success.*

16

Continuing the Journey

Pamela S. Dickerson, PhD, RN, NPDA-BC°, FAAN

Chapter 1 provided evidence to support the need for equity in nursing to better care for the populations we serve. Creating a more diverse nursing workforce provides opportunities for more efficiently and effectively addressing social determinants of health (SDOH), which significantly impact the health of Americans. Chapters 2 through 15 reflect the journeys of current nurse leaders who represent diverse backgrounds, cultures, and experiences. To continue the journey, individuals, academic providers from elementary school through graduate education, professional associations, employers, and government agencies must address areas of inequity and be proactive in supporting education, recruitment, retention, and promotion of nurses who can significantly contribute to quality health care. Lessons from the nurse leaders represented in this book can provide a framework for these efforts. Additional examples and opportunities are included in this chapter.

Many national nursing organizations have recently made commitments to address inequity in both patient care and the profession itself. Examples include but are not limited to the following:

- The American Nurses Association (ANA) has incorporated equity into its 2020–2023 strategic plan. Objective 3.5 speaks to addressing racism within the profession, and Objective 4.2

addresses the need to promote diversity, equity, and inclusion across the ANA Enterprise to support and role-model workplace practices that are culturally appropriate (ANA, 2020).

- The National Commission to Address Racism in Nursing was formed in 2021. The organization is comprised of 20 groups representing nursing practice and education across the country and is led by the ANA, the National Black Nurses Association, the National Coalition of Ethnic Minority Nurse Associations, and the National Association of Hispanic Nurses (ANA, 2021b). The vision of this group is that "the nursing profession exemplifies inclusivity, diversity, and equity, creating an antiracist praxis and environments" (ANA, 2021b, para. 8). Its mission is to establish standards of practice reflective of the work of nurses to address and mitigate systemic racism and the impact of racism on nurses and their practice.

- To support the work of the ANA Enterprise and the National Commission to Address Racism in Nursing, the updated *Nursing: Scope and Standards of Practice*, 4th ed. (ANA, 2021c) incorporates a standard specific to respectful and equitable practice. Expectations of nurses to address this standard include respect for individuals with differing worldviews; providing culturally appropriate care, including communication and support in decision making; advocating for policies that support health promotion for diverse individuals and groups; and developing processes to attain and maintain a diverse and multicultural workforce.

- Building on the ANA scope and standards, the Association for Nursing Professional Development (ANPD) revised its own *Nursing Professional Development: Scope and Standards of Practice* in 2022, similarly incorporating a standard for respectful and equitable practice (Harper & Maloney, 2022). Unique to the role of the nursing professional development (NPD) practitioner are expectations that NPD practitioners themselves will continue to learn and grow in the area of cultural humility, design education for nurses and other members of the healthcare team that reflect diversity in both learners and recipients of care, and work to achieve a more diverse NPD practitioner workforce.

The National Academy of Medicine has called on nursing to lead the transformation in contemporary health care to address inequities in care delivery, SDOH, and unique needs of individuals and families (National Academies of Sciences, Engineering, and Medicine [NASEM], 2021). Specific note is made of the fact that, to lead this transformation, nursing itself needs to be more reflective of the population it serves. As noted on page 9, "Building a diverse nursing workforce is a critical part of preparing nurses to address SDOH and health equity." Recommendations from the report include both individual initiatives and opportunities for academic and healthcare organizations to influence policy at regulatory, reimbursement, and governmental levels. These recommendations include:

- Efforts need to be made by national nursing organizations to develop shared agendas for addressing inequities and SDOH. Work by ANA, the National Commission to Address Racism in Nursing, and updates to the scope and standards for both nursing as a whole and NPD practitioners in particular reflect progress in addressing this recommendation.
- Actions to support nursing's efforts to address SDOH and health equity need to be addressed at organizational, governmental, and financial levels.

- Commitment is required from numerous organizations to provide evidence-based interventions to improve the health and well-being of nurses. This takes on particular importance in relation to the unique challenges of the COVID-19 pandemic and reflects the importance of nurses caring for themselves so they can effectively care for others.
- Barriers that interfere with nurses' abilities to practice to the full extent of their education must be removed, particularly in relation to addressing SDOH and inequities in care.
- Payment mechanisms to support the work of nurses in healthcare settings need to change, particularly in public health, school nursing, and other arenas that impact health equity.
- Nursing expertise must be included in efforts to creatively address SDOH and health equity challenges.
- Academic and continuing professional development curricula and activities must be developed to ensure that nurses are well positioned to address SDOH and health equity.
- The importance and value of the nursing workforce must be strengthened and protected, particularly when dealing with health emergencies, natural disasters, and climate change.
- A research agenda must be developed and implemented to assess the impact of nursing interventions on SDOH, health equity, and nurses' own health and well-being.

There are numerous ways nurses, individually and collectively, can contribute to achievement of these recommendations. As noted in Chapter 1, use of the nursing process can guide work in assessment, planning, implementation, and evaluation of efforts to achieve equity within the nursing profession and those it serves. The stories by nurse leaders in this book have illustrated their own journeys to address inequities in nursing education and practice

and the strides they have made in navigating change, both personally and professionally. Building on their examples, suggestions are
presented for consideration by individual nurses, nursing practice
and shared governance committees, nurse educators, nurse administrators, and others who impact nursing education and practice.
This includes academic educators and counselors from elementary
through high school as they encourage students, particularly those
from marginalized communities, to consider a career in nursing.

Developing and Supporting Career and Technical Education

Many school districts are increasing their focus on career development in elementary and middle schools, building curricula and creating opportunities for students to explore opportunities beyond
preparation for college. These efforts are predicated on evidence
that actively engaging younger students in what they are learning and how that learning impacts career opportunities leads to
better outcomes (Strom, 2019). This early focus on career opportunities is particularly important for students with limited financial
resources and limited awareness of opportunities available to them.

Career education can address specific areas of development,
like science or math, but also includes communication, teamwork, collaboration, and accountability. Encouraging students
to obtain industry-related credentials prior to graduation from
high school can help them obtain jobs to support living expenses,
attend college if desired, and begin building a work-related portfolio of achievements. Strom (2019) cautions, however, that focus on
career readiness upon high school graduation can widen the diversity gap by discouraging college attendance for those who enter the
workforce immediately.

The Association for Career and Technical Education published a guide in 2018 to support career exploration in middle school. Based on data showing that middle school is an optimal time for students to begin exploring career opportunities, the Association recommends integration of career and technical education (CTE) programming that allows middle school students to assess personal strengths and interests to empower them to select education tracks in "career clusters," preparing them for future employment opportunities. Specific recommendations include incorporating career-related learning and projects in classrooms, building skills important in the employment setting, maintaining flexibility as students explore options, using online tools to support academic and career planning, facilitating interactions with community leaders in various career roles, and providing opportunities for student participation in related career-development experiences.

The difference between traditional "vocational education" training and current approaches to CTE is striking. Gonser (2018) asserts that CTE programs are "uniquely positioned to prepare young adults for the future of work" (para. 3). The history of vocational programs to attract low-income and minority students is a deterrent to some, while others embrace the opportunity for new ways of looking at CTE. Data reported by Advance CTE (2020) show high graduation rates among high school students who participated in CTE programs. Further, over a 20-year period, more CTE learners completed college preparation courses than other students, and 86% of high school graduates who participated in CTE programs in 2004 subsequently enrolled in post-secondary education, with the majority of them earning degrees.

The federal Strengthening Career and Technical Education for the 21st Century Act (Perkins V), includes a reserve fund designed to support CTE programs as well as rural communities and those with performance disparities among community populations (Advance CTE, 2021). Working in conjunction with state goals to support high-skill and in-demand industries, the funds can be allocated to both high school and higher-level educational institutions. A survey conducted by Advance CTE (2021) identified equity as the highest prioritization in use of Perkins funds, followed by work-based learning.

As one specific example related to health care, Taylor (2018) describes a multifocal approach to increasing opportunities for healthcare careers, particularly among minority students in the Chicago area. One component of the program is a massive open online course (MOOC) developed by Northwestern University and integrated with the Chicago Public Schools' CTE curriculum. The course, Career 911: Your Future Job in Medicine and Health Care, introduces students to healthcare career opportunities. These educational experiences are combined with other initiatives, such as having medical students speak to high school students about their career journeys, offering shadowing or observational experiences in the healthcare environment, and creating mentoring opportunities that benefit both students and healthcare professionals. Taylor (2018) comments that limiting recruitment to high-performing students "weakens the health care career pipeline and perpetuates the existing trend of declining minority enrollment in medical school and graduate programs related to health care careers" and that "development of health care career programs that are strategically intentional about supporting minority students all the way through to career placement is profoundly requisite in paving a cogent pathway toward achieving diversity in the health care workforce" (p. 3).

As another example, Akron Children's Hospital in Akron, Ohio, has developed the "Career Launch" workforce diversity development program, designed to "provide current employees and community members with educational opportunities to start and advance their careers" (Akron Children's Hospital, 2020, p. 1). The program provides participants with a job at the hospital, in addition to benefits, tuition reimbursement, and additional financial resources. The program offers an opportunity for participants to build knowledge and skills in a supportive environment while continuing their academic progression. The hospital has partnered with community agencies and local colleges to enable participants to achieve degrees to be medical assistants, licensed practical nurses, respiratory therapists, and other healthcare team members. Career progression within the institution occurs as individuals continue to learn and grow.

Informally, resources also exist in children's literature and other sources to encourage diversity, equity, and inclusion. While not specifically related to health care, books such as these challenge young readers to think about equity and inclusion as a normal part of life experiences. One example is the book *Mary Wears What She Wants* by Keith Negley (2019). Young readers are encouraged to reflect on making choices based on changing the status quo— in Mary's case, by wearing pants instead of dresses. The story is derived from the experiences of Mary Edwards Walker, a female Civil War surgeon. Another is a picture book by Malala Yousafzai (2017) entitled *Malala's Magic Pencil*. The author uses her own lived experiences to illustrate how a young girl from Pakistan wishes she had a magic pencil to create the world of her dreams. She learns that she has the power to make change, including enabling girls to access academic education, with her own abilities, even without a magic pencil. Specific to nursing, Dr. Scharmaine Lawson, FNP-BC, PMHNP-BC, FAANP, FAAN, has created a children's book series entitled *NOLA the Nurse*. As Dr. Lawson notes on her website, "While there were a few books about nurses, there were none that encompassed the role I play, so I sought to create a diverse heroine that would pique my daughter's interest" (Lawson, n.d.). The series has grown to a global brand with 30 titles, and some have been translated into French and/or Spanish. A related animated project will be released soon. In a follow-up email, Dr. Lawson stated, "This shows that representation matters, and that ALL communities need to feel included when it comes to children's literature and nursing roles. The future of nursing is diverse, and we need to be intentional and creative about how we proceed" (S. Lawson, personal communication, January 19, 2022). Resources such as these stimulate children to believe in themselves, identify and work toward goals, and realize their unique potential.

Opportunities to Increase Equity in Nursing

The National Academy of Medicine, in its 2021 release of *The Future of Nursing 2020–2030*, addresses the need to transform nursing education. In particular, the study points out that the nursing profession currently does not reflect the diversity of the U.S. population (NASEM, 2021). More nurses of different cultural and ethnic backgrounds are needed in all areas of practice. There is double value in this goal—patients and families are more receptive to advice, education, and care from people who are most like them, and nurses of these different backgrounds can challenge students of their cultures to aspire to careers in nursing and health care. Nursing, because of its reach throughout the healthcare system, has a unique opportunity to provide leadership in both diversifying the profession and developing strategies to support population health.

Multiple opportunities exist for nurses to support equity in nursing practice—both from the standpoint of increasing diversity and inclusion within the nursing profession and in supporting equity in care that is provided for individuals, groups, and communities. The ANA's *Nursing: Scope and Standards of Practice*, 4th edition (2021c), incorporates a standard specific to respectful and equitable practice. Likewise, the *Nursing Professional Development Scope and Standards of Practice*, 4th edition (Harper & Maloney, 2022), includes a standard specific to social equity in NPD practice. The interprofessional practice and learning environments encompass aspects such as recruitment and retention, competency development and maintenance, and ongoing professional learning. There are specific ways nurses can use these standards to support social equity within the profession as well as in the provision of patient/family, group, or community health care:

- Individual nurses can act as advocates for nursing, and specifically for their own specialty areas of practice. In this role of advocate, nurses can investigate implementation of CTE programs in middle and high schools in their communities. If such programs exist, how can the nurse and the healthcare organization support CTE specific to healthcare career interest? Opportunities might include assistance in curriculum development, provision of examples and case studies to help students learn about career opportunities in health care, and shadowing/mentoring experiences for students as they consider career choices. If programs do not currently exist, how can the nurse and the healthcare organization facilitate their development?
- Nurses practicing in the academic setting have an opportunity to look at admission and retention policies, curriculum design, academic progression requirements, and other aspects of undergraduate and graduate nursing education programs to ensure that there is flexibility to meet the needs of learners

with diverse learning needs. Many of the nurse leaders who shared stories in this book reflected on challenges they faced as they applied to, entered, and progressed through their academic programs. How can the academic environment shift to a more welcoming and supporting environment to facilitate meeting individual learners' needs while upholding the quality and integrity of the academic program?

- Nurses in hospitals and community practice settings often have relationships with area schools/colleges of nursing as they facilitate student learning experiences. Conversations with leaders in the academic environment can include enrollment requirements for LPN, ADN, and/or baccalaureate programs. Are academic programs in the area structuring enrollment practices in such a way as to be socially equitable? Are there requirements in place that create barriers for those with low income, lack of proficiency in English language, socially disadvantaged backgrounds, or other challenges? How can barriers be removed or reduced to support successful matriculation and academic progression of all students interested in healthcare careers? Can the nurse serve as a mentor or advocate for those who might have difficulty with the academic curriculum due to language challenges, childcare/family issues, reluctance to self-advocate, or other issues?

- As nurses design, develop, and engage in learning experiences within the practice environment, opportunities exist to expand one's own education and that of colleagues related to cultural humility. Is the nurse selecting intentional educational experiences to facilitate personal and professional growth in the areas of cultural awareness, health literacy, and SDOH? The professional learning environment also creates a venue for exploring career opportunities in areas such as public health, school nursing, occupational health nursing, and other community-based practice settings that offer unique ways for nurses to address health equity challenges.

- In the healthcare practice environment, awareness of an individual's strengths and interest in career progression often becomes apparent. The department clerk might be interested in enrolling in an LPN program; the professional development associate might be interested in a degree in educational design. Nurses can assist individuals in accessing resources to help those dreams become reality. That might include exploring opportunities for scholarships, negotiating work time to allow for school attendance, and navigating barriers to academic program enrollment.

- Nurse administrators have an opportunity to examine workplace culture and opportunities for a diverse population of healthcare employees to thrive in the practice environment. Are hiring practices reflective of today's social climate? Are human resources staff working to recruit nurses representative of the populations served by the organization? Is there ongoing professional development for all nurses and other members of the healthcare team to learn about equity, cultural values and norms that impact health care, and SDOH factors that influence patient/family decisions, care, and health outcomes? How are future nurse leaders identified and mentored? Many of the nurse leaders' stories included in this book reflect their initial reluctance to embark on leadership progression because of cultural norms, fear of failure, or concern about the leadership selection process, which might not value their expertise or select the individual to fill a "quota" rather than based on competencies for the role. How are potential leaders supported in their professional growth, regardless of their skin color, hairstyle, gender, or accent?

- Nurse researchers have a unique opportunity to examine how current and upcoming changes will impact health equity, both in terms of workforce diversity and public health outcomes. As noted by Cohen et al. (2021), the nursing health services research agenda for 2020–2030 includes five focal areas: improving access to and effectiveness of behavioral health interventions and services, improving access to and effectiveness of primary health care and systems, improving maternal healthcare outcomes and the delivery of maternal health care, improving care provided to older adults, and controlling healthcare costs while demonstrating the value of nursing's contributions to care. Key issues influencing these research priorities were the fact that nurses are primarily prepared for acute-care practice and not community-based practice and the need to "develop a diverse nurse workforce with the knowledge, skills, and competencies and cultural humility to serve an increasingly diverse public" (Cohen et al., 2021, p. 271).
- In the broader community setting, nurses have an opportunity to be a voice and an influencing power related to social equity. Participating in community groups, running for municipal office or serving on a school board, and offering to speak to school groups about health careers are specific ways the nurse can share messages of equitable health promotion, while also encouraging individuals from diverse backgrounds to consider nursing and/or other health-related careers.
- While nursing is consistently recognized as a highly trusted profession (Saad, 2020), nursing's voice is often not heard in the public venue. Nurses who enjoy writing might consider

authoring children's books such as those described above that show diversity in employees and careers in health care. They can seek elected office at state or national levels, can offer to serve as panelists on community forums related to social equity, and can engage with groups supporting opportunity and advancement for all citizens, regardless of race, cultural background, social situation, or financial status.

Health Equity and Innovation in Nursing

A common theme among the stories included in this book is a lack of encouragement to challenge the status quo with innovative approaches to care delivery and change in processes. Frequently, they were told to focus on tasks, had their qualifications questioned, and were told, "Do what you are told." They continued to seek challenges in diverse settings and succeeded. This is not unique to these individuals. Their gender, ethnicity, race, and cultural identity did not stop them from pursuing health equity and innovation as nursing leaders.

The impact of technology in health care is reflected in some of their stories and provides an avenue for diverse nurses to innovate and lead in the future. The September 2021 edition of *The Online Journal of Issues in Nursing* (*OJIN*) provides a detailed blueprint for nurses to advance technology in health care using innovative approaches that will promote health equity (McGrow, 2021). Here are some examples for all nurses to consider as they move out of the box of "we've always done it this way" to embrace the challenges of innovation in nursing:

- The nurse leaders profiled here pursued higher education as a pathway to achievement. Formal education is available for nurse informaticists and must be supplemented with a support system of mentorship. Building a network is essential for professional growth and learning from peers. Like our leaders demonstrate, gaining confidence and building competencies is valuable, as is being engaged in professional organizations (Backonja et al., 2021).

- Our nurse leaders understand the importance of supporting nurses' practice needs. Use of artificial intelligence (AI) is an opportunity to apply data to address complex clinical questions and improve patient care. Nurses must be involved in the design of AI solutions to ensure that bias and potential inequities are addressed and health equity is promoted. Nurses' input and collaboration with technology developers and interprofessional teams will ensure that projects for safety initiatives and quality improvement projects address patient care issues (Tiase & Cato, 2021).

- Several of our nurse leaders have been integral to successful implementation of innovations to improve practice and education. Nurses throughout history have been innovators. Hackathons, innovation incubators, and innovation accelerators are three methods for nurses to use an innovation and design thinking framework to add value to healthcare practice and education. Nurse-led hackathons with other collaborators form teams guided by mentors, develop problem statements, create a prototype, and test solutions over a two-day period. The background, problem, and solution are presented to a panel of expert stakeholders for resolution. Innovation incubators take an early-stage idea and develop it with testing and research. An example of a nurse-led innovation incubator is the Center for Innovations in Care Delivery in Boston, which influences practice by recognizing gaps and inefficiencies in care delivery and identifying opportunities for improvements in care and services. Innovation accelerators are educational opportunities tied to funding and mentorship for innovative ideas (Kagan et al., 2021).

- Our nurse leaders are aware of the importance of big data in nursing. Nurse scholars have focused on the practice setting, and there is still a need for emphasis on data competencies. Nurse faculty must prepare students with knowledge and skills about statistics, programming, and informatics. There is a need to apply big data approaches to enhance the mission of nursing and quality patient outcomes. A diverse nursing workforce must operationalize and integrate big data in nursing practice, research, education, and policy (Carter-Templeton et al., 2021).

These four examples illustrate application of the words of one of our nurse leaders, Dr. Ernest Grant, in Chapter 7: "We need to incorporate more innovation and technology that will allow nurses to work smarter, more efficiently, and still be able to provide that much needed hands-on care."

Summary

Appreciating and valuing the stories of nurse leaders who have contributed to this book provides opportunities for nurses and others to significantly impact the profession by increasing diversity in nursing and improving quality care that reflects the diversity and unique needs of the patient populations nursing serves.

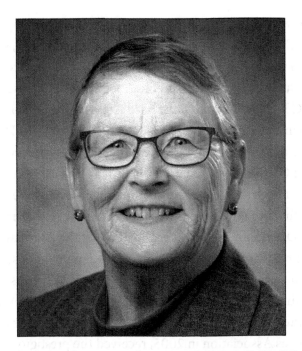

Pamela S. Dickerson, PhD, RN, NPDA-BC®, FAAN
Nursing Professional Development Specialist

Dr. Dickerson has been actively engaged in the practice of nursing for over 40 years and involved in continuing education for health-care professionals since the mid-1980s. The focus of her work relates to developing, implementing, and evaluating educational activities to achieve quality outcomes in professional practice and delivery of care. In her most recent role, she served as director of professional development for the Montana Nurses Association, with accountability for MNA's accredited approver and provider units. Dr. Dickerson is originally a graduate of a diploma school of nursing and has earned baccalaureate and master's degrees in nursing and a doctorate in health administration. She has been actively involved with the American Nurses Credentialing Center's (ANCC) Commission on Accreditation since 1995, where she has served as commissioner, appraiser for primary accreditation, and surveyor for joint accreditation. She currently serves as an ANCC NCPD Commissioner and Accreditation Review Committee member for the Joint Accreditation program. Dr. Dickerson serves as an editorial board member and peer reviewer for the Journal of Continuing Education in Nursing and is the author of numerous articles in peer-reviewed nursing journals. She is the editor of the fifth edition of the Core Curriculum for Nursing Professional Development, published in 2017 by the Association for Nursing Professional Development. She is a member of several professional associations, including the American Nurses Association and the Association for Nurses in Professional Development. She was inducted into the Cornelius Leadership Congress of the Ohio Nurses Association in 2005, received the prestigious ANCC President's Award in 2010, and was inducted as a fellow in the American Academy of Nursing in 2013. In 2021, she received the Marlene Kramer Award from the Association for Nursing Professional Development, recognizing her lifetime commitment to and leadership in nursing professional development.

REFERENCES

Advance CTE. (2020). *Career technical education and learner achievement.* https://cte.careertech.org/sites/default/files/documents/fact-sheets/CTE_a/nd_student_achievement_2020_0.pdf

Advance CTE. (2021). *Strengthening career and technical education for the 21st century act* (Perkins V). https://cte.careertech.org/sites/default/files/documents/fact-sheets/Perkins_V_Reserve_Fund_2021.pdf

Akron Children's Hospital. (2020). *Career launch.* https://careers.akronchildrens.org/career-launch

American Association of Colleges of Nursing. (2019). *Enhancing diversity fact sheet.* https://www.aacnnursing.org/Portals/42/News/Factsheets/Enhancing-Diversity-Factsheet.pdf

American Association of Colleges of Nursing. (2021). *The essentials: Core competencies for professional nursing education.* https://www.aacnnursing.org/Portals/42/AcademicNursing/pdf/Essentials-2021.pdf

American History Today. (n.d.). *Melting pot.* https://www.americanhistoryusa.com/topic/melting-pot/

American Institute of Stress. (n.d.). *The Holmes-Rahe stress inventory.* https://www.stress.org/holmes-rahe-stress-inventory

American Nurses Association. (2020). *2020–2023 strategic plan.* https://www.nursingworld.org/ana-enterprise/about-us/anae-strategic-plan-2020---2023

American Nurses Association. (2021a). *Advanced practice registered nurse.* https://nursingworld.org/practice-policy/workforce/what-is-nursing/aprn

American Nurses Association. (2021b). *National Commission to Address Racism in Nursing.* https://www.nursingworld.org/practice-policy/workforce/clinical-practice-material/national-commission-to-address-racism-in-nursing/

American Nurses Association. (2021c). *Nursing: Scope and standards of practice* (4th ed.).

Association for Career and Technical Education. (2018). *Career exploration in middle school: Setting students on the path to success.* https://www.acteonline.org/wp-content/uploads/2018/02/ACTE_CC_Paper_FINAL.pdf

Association of American Medical Colleges. (n.d.). *Applying to medical school as an international applicant.* https://students-residents.aamc.org/applying-medical-school/applying-medical-school-international-applicant

Backonja, U., Mook, P., & Langford, L. (2021). Calling nursing informatics leaders: Opportunity for personal and professional growth. *Online Journal of Issues in Nursing, 26*(3), Article 6. https://doi.org/10.3912/OJIN.Vol26No03Man06

Baldwin, J. (2017). Culture, prejudice, racism, and discrimination. In *Oxford research encyclopedia of communication.* https://doi.org/10.1093/acrefore/9780190228613.013.164

Baldwin, J., Lowe, J., Brooks, J., Charbonneau-Dahlen, B., Lawrence, G., Johnson-Jennings, M., Padgett, G., Kelley, M., & Camplain, C. (2020). Formative research and cultural tailoring of a substance abuse prevention program for American Indian youth: Findings from the Intertribal Talking Circle Intervention. *Health Promotion Practice, 22*(6), 778–785. https://doi.org/10.1177/1524839920918551

Book Series in Order. (n.d.). *Cherry Ames books in order.* www.bookseriesinorder.com/cherry-ames/

Carter-Templeton, H., Nicoll, L., Wrigley, J., & Wyatt, T. (2021). Big data in nursing: A bibliometric analysis. *Online Journal of Issues in Nursing, 26*(3), Article 2. https://doi.org/10.3912/OJIN.Vol26No03Man02

Christian, L., Cater, G., Dieujuste, C. (2021). The Dotson Bridge and Mentoring Program: A success story. *Nurse Educator, 46*(5), 306–310. https://doi.org/10.1097/NNE.0000000000000958

Clark, N. (Ed.). (2015, June 2). *Education in Kenya-wenr.* WENR. https://wenr.wes.org/2015/06/education-kenya

Cohen, C. C., Barnes, H., Buerhaus, P. I., Martsolf, G. R., Clarke, S. P., Konelan, K., & Tubbs-Cooley, H. L. (2021). Top priorities for the next decade of nursing health services research. *Nursing Outlook, 69*(3), 265–275. https://doi.org/10.1016/j.outlook.2020.12.004

Cook, E. (1913a). *The life of Florence Nightingale* (Vol. 1). Macmillan.

Cook, E. (1913b). *The life of Florence Nightingale* (Vol. 2). Macmillan.

Current Nursing. (2020). *Orlando's nursing process theory.* https://www.currentnursing.com/nursing_theory/Orlando_nursing_process.html

Donahue, M. P. (2011). *Nursing: The finest art* (3rd ed.). Mosby.

Dossey, B., Selanders, L., Beck, D., & Attewell, A. (2005). *Florence Nightingale today: Healing, leadership, global action.* American Nurses Association.

Durant, W. (1926). *The story of philosophy.* Simon & Schuster.

Equitable Evaluation Initiative. (2020). *Why the equitable evaluation framework?* https://www.equitableeval.org/why-ee

Equity Literacy Institute. (2021). *Equity assessment.* https://www.equityliteracy.org/equity-assessment

Falker, A. (2021). *Implicit and explicit bias: Where do we go from here?* Academy of Medical-Surgical Nurses. https://amsn.org/publications/amsn-blog/implicit-and-explicit-bias

Gonser, S. (2018). Revamped and rigorous, career and technical education is ready to be taken seriously. *Hechinger Report.* https://hechingerreport.org/revamped-and-rigorous-career-and-technical-education-is-ready-to-be-taken-seriously/

Gretter, L. (1893). *Florence Nightingale pledge.* https://nursing.vanderbilt.edu/news/florence-nightingale-pledge/

Harper, M., & Maloney, P. (Eds.). (2022). *Nursing professional development: Scope and standards of practice* (4th ed.). Association for Nursing Professional Development.

Health Policy Institute of Ohio. (2020). *COVID-19 minority health strike force blueprint.* https://coronavirus.ohio.gov/static/MHSF/MHSF-Blueprint.pdf

Institute of Medicine. (1999). *To err is human: Building a safer health system.* National Academies Press. https://doi.org/10.17226/9728

Institute of Medicine. (2001). *Crossing the quality chasm: A new health system for the 21st century.* National Academies Press. https://doi.org/10.17226/10027

Institute of Medicine. (2011). *The future of nursing: Leading change, advancing health.* National Academies Press. https://doi.org/10.17226/12956

Johnson, S. (2016). *Nightingale's legacy: The evolution of American nurse leaders.* American Nurses Association.

Johnson & Johnson. (2016). *The Johnson and Johnson campaign for nursing's future celebrates 14 years.* https://nursing.jnj.com/the-johnson-johnson-i-campaign-for-nursings-future-i-celebrates-fourteen-years

Kagan, O., Littlejohn, J., Nadel, H., & Leary, M. (2021). Evolution of nurse-led hackathons, incubators, and accelerators from an innovation ecosystem perspective. *Online Journal of Issues in Nursing, 26*(3), Article 3. https://doi.org/10.3912/OJIN.Vol26No03Man03

Kaini, B. K. (2017). *Interprofessional team collaboration in health care.* https://globaljournals.org/GJMR_Volume17-1-Interprofessional-Team-Collaboration.pdf

Kliewer, A., Mahmud, M., & Wayland, B. (n.d.). *"Kill the Indian; Save the man":
Remembering the stories of Indian boarding schools.* Gaylord College of Journalism

and Mass Communications. https://www.ou.edu/gaylord/exiled-to-indian-country/content/remembering-the-stories-of-indian-boarding-schools

Lawson, S. (n.d.). *NOLA the nurse*. https://nolathenurse.com

Legacy.com. (2005). *Henrieta Villeascusa obituary*. https://www.legacy.com/obituaries/pasadenastarnews/obituary.aspx?pid=3263612

Library of Congress. (n.d.). *Project on the decade of the brain*. www.loc.gov/loc/brain/

Lowe, J. (2002). Cherokee self-reliance. *Journal of Transcultural Nursing, 13*(4), 287–295. https://doi.org/10.1177/104365902236703

Lowe, J., & Crow, K. (2009). Utilization of a Native American conceptual framework to transform nursing education. *International Journal for Human Caring, 13*(3), 56–64. https://search.informit.org/doi/10.3316/ielapa.285541468166522

Lowe, J., Liang, H., & Henson, J. (2016). Preventing substance use among Native American early adolescents. *Journal of Community Psychology, 44*(8), 997–1010. https://doi.org/10.1002/jcop.21823

Lowe, J., & Struthers, R. (2001). A conceptual framework of nursing in Native American culture. *Journal of Nursing Scholarship, 33*(3), 279–283. https://doi.org/10.1111/j.1547-5069.2001.00279.x

Lowe, J., Wagner, E., Hospital, M. M., Morris, S. L., Thompson, M., Sawant, M., Kelley, M., & Millender, M. (2019). Utility of the Native-reliance theoretical framework, model, and questionnaire. *Journal of Cultural Diversity, 26*(2), 61–68.

Masselink, L., & Jones, C. (2014). Immigration policy and internationally educated nurses in the United States: A brief history. *Nursing Outlook, 62*(1), 39–45. https://doi.org/10.1016/j.outlook.2013.10.012

McGrow, K. (2021). Advancing technology in healthcare: Are you on board? *Online Journal of Issues in Nursing, 26*(3). https://doi.org/10.3912/OJIN.Vol26No03ManOS

Mt. Vernon Register News. (1966, March 26). *King charges Negro medical care inferior*. Associated Press.

National Academies of Science, Engineering, and Medicine. (2021). *The future of nursing 2020–2030: Charting a path to achieve health equity*. National Academies Press. https://doi.org/10.17226/25982

National Association of Hispanic Nurses. (2021). *Henrieta Villaescusa, MPH, RN*. https://nahnnet.org/about/bios/Henrieta-Villaescusa

National League for Nursing. (2019). *A vision for the integration of the social determinants of health into nursing education curricula*. https://www.nln.org/

docs/default-source/uploadedfiles/default-document-library/social-determinants-of-health.pdf?sfvrsn=aa66a50d_0

Negley, K. (2019). *Mary wears what she wants*. Children's Library Lady. https://childrenslibrarylady.com/mary-wears-what-she-wants

Negotiation Experts. (n.d.). *BATNA*. https://www.negotiations.com/definition/batna

The Ohio State University College of Public Health. (2020). *Ohio's COVID-19 population needs assessment: Minimizing the disparate impact of the pandemic and building foundations for health equity*. https://cph.osu.edu/sites/default/files/docs/covid19inequities/1-Full%20Report.pdf

Pukui, M. K. (1983). *'Ōlelo No'eau: Hawaiian proverbs & poetical sayings*. Honolulu: Bishop Museum Press.

Richards, L. (1911). *Reminiscences of Linda Richards, America's first trained nurse*. Thomas Tod Company.

Ross, L., Wood, S., Burgy, D., Eley, C., Guerra, M., Howard, T., Ledesma, E., Mitra, A., Ochoa, M., Perkins, A., Stowell, C., & Vazquez, M. (2019). *Planning for equity policy guide*. American Planning Association. https://www.planning.org/publications/document/9178541/

Saad, L. (2020). *U.S. ethics ratings rise for medical workers and teachers*. Gallup. https://gallup.com/poll/328136/ethics-rations-rise-medical-workers-teachers.aspx

Smiley, R., Ruttinger, C., Oliveira, C., Hudson, L., Allgeyer, R., Reneau, K., Silvistre, J., & Alexander, M. (2021). The 2020 national nursing workforce survey. *Journal of Nursing Regulation, 12*(Suppl.), S1–S16. https://doi.org/10.1016/S2155-8256(21)00027-2

Strom, S. (2019). What does 'career readiness' look like in middle school? *Hechinger Report*. https://www.hechingerreport.org/what-does-career-readiness-look-like-in-middle-school/

Taylor, S. (2018). The health care career pipeline: A program director's reflection on extending the resources of the university to the minority student community. *National Academy of Medicine*. https://doi.org/10.31478/201803b

Tiase, V., & Cato, K. (2021). From artificial intelligence to augmented intelligence: Practical guidance for nurses. *Online Journal of Issues in Nursing, 26*(3), Article 4. https://doi.org/10.3912/OJIN.Vol26No03Man04

U.S. Census Bureau. (2021a). *Racial and ethnic diversity in the United States: 2010 census and 2020 census*. https://www.census.gov/library/visualizations/interactive/racial-and-ethnic-diversity-in-the-united-states-2010-and-2020-census.html

U.S. Census Bureau. (2021b). *Sexual orientation and gender identity in the household pulse survey.* https://www.census.gov/library/visualizations/interactive/sexual-orientation-and-gender-identity.html

U.S. Citizenship and Immigration Services. (2020, August 13). *Students and employment.* https://www.uscis.gov/working-in-the-united-states/students-and-exchange-visitors/students-and-employment

U.S. News and World Report. (n.d.). *National liberal arts colleges rankings.* https://www.usnews.com/best-colleges/rankings/national-liberal-arts-colleges?schoolName=Ohio+Wesleyan+University

Western Governors University. (2019). *Minorities in nursing: Improving workforce diversity.* https://www.wgu.edu/blog/minorities-nursing-improving-workforce-diversity1901.html

Whiteman, K., Yaglowski, J., & Stephens, K. (2021). Critical thinking tools for quality improvement projects. *Critical Care Nurse, 41*(2), e1–e9. https://pubmed.ncbi.nlm.nih.gov/33791767/

Woo, B., DuMont, K., & Metz, A. (2019). *Equity at the center of implementation.* Center for the Study of Social Policy. https://cssp.org/2019/12/implementation-equity/

Woolforde, L. (2018). Nursing professional development: Our spheres of expansion. *Journal for Nurses in Professional Development, 34*(4), 237–238. https://doi.org/10.1097/NND.0000000000000457

World Health Organization. (2020). *Year of the nurse and the midwife 2020.* https://www.who.int/campaigns/annual-theme/year-of-the-nurse-and-the-midwife-2020

Yousafzai, M. (2017). *Malala's magic pencil.* Little, Brown Books for Young Readers. https://www.itseyeris.com/book/malala-s-magic-pencil